Social Aspects of Aids

for Daniel —
Jan '89
with love
Erica

Social Aspects of Aids

Edited by

Peter Aggleton and Hilary Homans

The Falmer Press
(A member of the Taylor & Francis Group)
London, New York and Philadelphia.

UK   The Falmer Press, Falmer House, Barcombe, Lewes, East Sussex, BN8 5DL

USA   The Falmer Press, Taylor & Francis Inc., 242 Cherry Street, Philadelphia, PA 19106-1906

First published 1988

Library of Congress Cataloguing in Publication Data is available on request

ISBN 1 85000 363 7
ISBN 1 85000 364 5 (pbk)

Jacket design by Caroline Archer

Printed in Great Britain by Taylor & Francis (Printers) Ltd, Basingstoke

Contents

Acknowledgements

The chapter 'Love in a cold climate' by Jeffrey Weeks was originally published in *Marxism Today*, 31, 1, pp. 12–17. The chapter 'Visual AIDS — Advertising ignorance' by Simon Watney was originally published in *New Socialist*, 47, pp 19–21. Both of these chapters are reproduced with the permission of their original publishers.

Preface

In October 1986 we jointly organized the first UK Conference on Social Aspects of AIDS at Bristol Polytechnic. This brought together a wide range of social researchers, health workers and others interested in developing a more critical appreciation of the social dynamics surrounding HIV infection and AIDS. This book contains a number of papers given at that conference but also contains a number of new contributions. We have also taken the opportunity of reprinting two articles from the growing literature on social aspects of AIDS which were originally published elsewhere.

We would like to thank our colleagues at Bristol Polytechnic for their support over the past year and owe a special debt to Helen Thomas for her work in preparing the manuscript for publication.

Peter Aggleton and **Hilary Homans**
October 1987

Introduction

Peter Aggleton and Hilary Homans

In June 1981, the Centers for Disease Control (CDC) in Atlanta, Georgia, began to receive its first reports of young men infected by what had until then been a relatively rare form of pneumonia — Pneumocystis carinii pneumonia (PCP). Simultaneously, reports were also received of an increased incidence of a hitherto rare form of skin tumour — Kaposi's sarcoma (KS) — also amongst men in their thirties and forties. Prior to this, both PCP and KS had been rare except amongst those whose immune systems had been weakened in some way. PCP, for example, had been common amongst those liberated from concentration camps at the end of the Second World War, and the incidence of Kaposi's sarcoma had hitherto been largely confined to elderly men in southern Europe and those living in rural areas of Central Africa. But two things made these new outbreaks of PCP and KS particularly significant. First, most of those affected seemed to be gay men. Second, the course of infection seemed to be much more severe than had hitherto been recorded. Many died or were severely debilitated within twelve months of their initial diagnosis.

For some time prior to this, physicians working in San Francisco, New York and other large American cities had begun to encounter otherwise healthy gay men with persistently swollen lymph nodes — Persistent Generalized Lymphadenopathy or Lymphadenopathy Syndrome — or who had fallen prey to one of a number of opportunistic infections caused by protozoa such as Toxoplasma gondii, bacteria such as Mycobacterium avium-intracellulare, viruses such as Cytomegalovirus and fungi such as Cryptococcus neoformans. In the case of people with Persistent Generalized Lymphadenopathy, the prognosis seemed at first relatively benign. Whilst some went on to develop opportunistic infections, the majority remained otherwise healthy for months and even years after being first diagnosed. But for those who developed opportunistic protozoal, bacterial, viral and fungal infections the future looked rather more bleak. Many failed to respond as expected to conventional forms of treatment or suffered unusually debilitating side-effects. Others experienced repeated bouts of opportunistic infection and often died.

In late 1981, a series of articles was published in the *New England Journal of Medicine* linking these opportunistic infections to identifiable changes in the functioning of the immune system. Many of those affected showed a marked depletion of a particular sub-set of white blood cells (T lymphocytes carrying the T4 surface marker). At about the same time, the first cases of PCP were diagnosed amongst heterosexual intravenous drug users in New York as well as amongst members of the Haitian community living in Miami and Brooklyn.

In 1982, the Centers for Disease Control coined the term Acquired Immune Deficiency Syndrome (AIDS) to describe,

> ... A reliably diagnosed disease that is at least moderately predictive of a defect in cell-mediated immunity, occurring in a person with no known cause of diminished resistance to disease. Such diseases include KS, PCP and other serious opportunistic infections ...

Thereafter, the scientific and medical establishment began to turn its attention to identifying the cause or causes of this immune defect. Initially, attention was focussed on the possibility that AIDS might be caused by a *single agent* — perhaps an already identified virus such as Cytomegalovirus or Epstein-Barr virus. Attention then shifted to the possibility that lifestyle variables might be the cause of immune breakdown. Early analyses using case-control interviews and regression analysis suggested that amongst gay men at least, those with AIDS could be reliably differentiated from others in terms of their number of sexual partners, the past history of infection by sexually transmitted diseases, their preference for particular forms of sexual expression (including receptive anal intercourse) and their recreational use of inhalants such as amyl and butyl nitrite. For a time, single viral explanations were superceded by those which emphasized the possibility that immune overload might be the cause of AIDS — occasioned perhaps by particular 'fast lane' lifestyles. As will be shown later in this book, this latter mode of explanation was influential in establishing from early on in the epidemic a moral agenda suggesting that AIDS might be a 'natural' consequence of 'unregulated sexual desire'.

In spring 1982, PCP was diagnosed in haemophiliacs who had

received Factor VIII blood centrates as part of their treatment. Shortly afterwards, opportunistic infections including PCP were diagnosed in people who had been the recipients of blood transfusions. These observations raised once more the possibility that a blood borne viral agent might be involved in the etiology of AIDS.

In late 1983, a retrovirus with an affinity for T-lymphocytes was isolated from a person with PGL in France and in early 1984 a similar virus was identified in People with AIDS (PWA) in the United States. These events gave new impetus to single agent viral explanations of AIDS. The viruses isolated — originally called Lymphadenopathy Virus (LAV) and Human T-cell Lymphotropic Virus Type III (HTLV-III), but subsequently renamed as Human Immunodeficiency Virus (HIV) — have since been shown to be similar, if not identical, in their structure.

Currently, there is widespread acceptance within the medical community and elsewhere concerning the central role with HIV plays in the etiology of AIDS — indeed the definition of AIDS offered by the Centers for Diseases Control was modified in August 1985 to include specific reference to HIV. It is also believed that the major means by which HIV is transmitted include blood, untreated blood products, semen, cervical and vaginal secretions and possibly breast milk. Whilst the virus has been isolated from saliva and tears, there is no evidence for transmissions by either of these routes. Tests have been developed to detect antibodies to this virus but there is currently considerable debate about both the manner in which the results they give should be interpreted and the uses to which the tests themselves should be put.

There continues to be controversy, however, about the role that lifestyle variables, intercurrent infection and life events such as pregnancy may play in determining whether or not a person with HIV infection subsequently develops AIDS. Certainly it is now known that AIDS is only one of a variety of consequences that can occur in the five to six-year period after HIV infection has been diagnosed. Other outcomes include relatively symptomless conditions, Persistent Generalized Lymphadenopathy and AIDS-Related Complex.

It is important to recognize that a minority of researchers continue to display some scepticism about the role played by HIV in the etiology of AIDS. Whilst in Europe and North America, clear attempts have been made to establish the hegemony of explanations which ascribe primacy to HIV in the causation of AIDS, claims contrary to such a view are still expressed. Some researchers have suggested that HIV may be a necessary but not sufficient cause of AIDS. Others have put forward the view that HIV may itself be an opportunist — a marker of infection by an as yet unidentified 'real' causal agent. According to the New York-based gay newspaper *New York Native* candidates for this 'real' causal agent include a DNA virus recently isolated from People with AIDS, African Swine Fever virus and untreated syphilitic infection.

The Social Dimensions of AIDS

But AIDS is not purely a biomedical phenomenon — it has important social dimensions as well. These range from the psychological consequences of being medically diagnosed as either HIV antibody positive or as having AIDS to the complex social processes that organize popular perceptions and social responses to AIDS (Altman, 1986).

Social researchers of all persuasions have an interest in AIDS. For some, AIDS may simply be another disease with a social epidemiology that needs to be mapped and with economic costs that need to be assessed. Others have seen in AIDS the chance to lay claim to much needed research funding to explore, amongst other things, the diversity of human sexual practice. A few have probed beneath the surface of popular responses to AIDS to identify the dynamics of racism, erotophobia, homophobia and heterosexism at work within them. For yet others, AIDS has provided a case study of the ways in which a medical category can be used to give new impetus to the reproduction and transformation of old social divisions — between gay and non-gay people, between black and white, between young and old, between prostitutes and their clients and between injecting drug users and others.

This book contains a selection of the papers which were originally written for the first UK Conference on Social Aspects of AIDS held at Bristol Polytechnic in October 1986. To these we have added a number of other contributions which help map out the main areas of research interest in Britain at the time. Whilst social enquiry relating to AIDS is still in its infancy, it is possible to identify in the following chapters a number of themes which will undoubtedly be influential in helping establish the agenda for future research into the social aspects of AIDS.

The first of these themes relates to a general concern amongst social researchers working in this field to identify the complexity (as well as the enormity) of the task that confronts them. In this respect, Jeffrey Weeks' opening chapter '*Love in a cold climate*' provides a useful introduction to the range of social and political issues that AIDS raises. By addressing the symbolic functions which AIDS serves, and by locating an analysis of these within the context of more general moves to secure a new and repressive moralism, Weeks begins an exploration of a central paradox created by the AIDS health crisis — that in the midst of moral panic and popular prejudice there have been unheralded degrees of commitment, courage and responsibility. Which of these two opposing forces wins out in the end will be central in influencing not only the future course of the epidemic, but also the quality of much of our social life.

Ken Plummer's chapter *'Organizing AIDS'* is a sophisticated and carefully argued attempt to identify the range of issues which need to be addressed in future research into social aspects of AIDS. He begins his analysis by identifying some of the key social meanings which AIDS has engendered. He then explores some of the ways in which AIDS has been linguistically organized — through the discourse of medicalization and stigma; publically organized — through moral panic and the scapegoating of apparently 'guilty victims'; personally organized — through the responses that PWAs and others have made; and socially organized — at the level of community responses and changes in gay sexuality. Plummer is not overly optimistic about the future course of events, but sees some positive potential in the responses of those who have been most affected by the epidemic.

Simon Watney's first chapter *'AIDS, "moral panic" theory and homophobia'* begins by analyzing some of the ways in which AIDS has been represented in the British popular press. He is highly critical of the speed with which AIDS came to be represented as a 'gay plague' as well as the alacrity with which so-called 'innocent' and 'guilty' victims of the disease have to be identified. For Watney, AIDS has become a 'powerful condensor for a great range of social, sexual and psychic anxieties'. Hence the intensity of the struggle to define what the syndrome is 'with the virus being used by all and sundry as a kind of glove puppet from the mouth of which different interest groups speak their values'. Central to an understanding of social uses to which AIDS has been put is an appreciation of the ways in which 'AIDS has been mobilized to embody a variety of perceived threats to individual and social stability, organized around the spectacle of illicit sex and physical corruption'. AIDS has been used above all to 'stabilize the figure of the heterosexual family unit ... with which individuals are endlessly invited to identify their collective interests and their very core of being'.

Keith Alcorn's contribution *'Illness, metaphor and AIDS'* pursues a related line of argument to this, but explores more specifically the social uses to which AIDS has been put as a 'disease of lifestyle', an 'illness of difference'. He also identifies some of the ways in which AIDS has been used as a vehicle by which to further individualize responsibility for health care in Britain, but sees hope in the impetus which AIDS has given to alternative and complementary styles of health care intervention.

Kaye Wellings' chapter '*Perceptions of risk: Media treatments of AIDS*' continues this exploration of the ways in which AIDS has been represented via an analysis of early newspaper reporting of the syndrome. Her particular interest lies in identifying the implications of media representations of AIDS for popular perceptions of risk. She examines a series of disturbing discontinuities and contradictions in 'quality' and 'popular' newspaper accounts of AIDS between 1983 and 1985. Her analysis focusses in particular on the systematic mis-reporting of *who* is most affected, *how many* are affected, what the *causes* of AIDS are and how the disease is *transmitted*.

Media representations of AIDS are likely to be particularly powerful in influencing the lay beliefs about AIDS that people share. Some of these are explored in Ian Warwick, Peter Aggleton and Hilary Homans' chapter on '*Young people's beliefs about AIDS*'. Their research confirms the view that lay beliefs about health and illness frequently co-exist alongside modern bio-medical explanations. With respect to AIDS, and in spite of recent government public information campaigns, young people continue to subscribe to miasmatic, endogenous, serendipitous and retributionist lay beliefs about its origins and modes of transmission. These may be influential in disorientating the impact of conventional approaches to health education which rely on information-giving as a strategy by which to encourage behavioural change.

The four remaining chapters in this book focus upon a range of relatively diverse issues currently of interest to social researchers. Tony Coxon's chapter '*The numbers game: The "gay lifestyle", epidemiology of AIDS and social science*' discusses some of the difficulties associated with predicting the future incidence of HIV infection. It critically examines the research methods that epidemiologists and others have hitherto used in their attempts to gain baseline estimates of the prevalence of 'high risk' sexual acts. Without accurate estimates of these, it is impossible to build statistical models by which to estimate the future course of the epidemic. Coxon reports on findings from his own research into gay lifestyles which uses a variety of enquiry methods to triangulate upon the acts in question.

The following two chapters explore some of the practical steps that have been taken to enhance public awareness about AIDS. Hugh Robertson's chapter '*AIDS: A trade union issue*' identifies some of the different responses that British trade unions have made to AIDS. He identifies a significant contrast between the actions of trade unions which have seen AIDS as a health and safety issue and those which have seen it as an equal opportunities concern.

Hilary Homans and Peter Aggleton in their chapter '*Health education, HIV infection and AIDS*' identify a series of paradigms or models of health education within which AIDS education can take place. In their analysis of health education practice in Britain and elsewhere, they contrast information-giving approaches to AIDS education with those that share a commitment to more participatory forms of learning. They review the goals and likely outcomes of these alternative strategies, which include self-empowerment, community-oriented and socially transformatory models of health education.

In the final chapter in this book '*Visual AIDS; Advertising ignorance*' Simon Watney critically examines aspects of the public information campaign that was launched, to widespread popular acclaim, by the UK government in early 1987.

Some Recurring Themes

Throughout the chapters that this book contains a number of themes recur. Central among these is the extent to which popular and professional understandings of AIDS have been informed by racism, homophobia and heterosexism. In the light of the analyses presented here, there can be little doubt that these divisive structures have played a critical role in establishing moral and political agendas around AIDS which seek to further stigmatize and pathologize those who already occupy marginal positions in society. Of particular concern in this respect is the speed with which AIDS has been 'captured' for the reconstruction of moral imperatives which seek to privilege above all other forms of sexual expression those that are narrowly focussed upon procreative and penetrative vaginal intercourse relationships within the context of exclusive and life-long monogamous relationships.

A not unrelated theme to this, examines the processes by which AIDS has been progressively individualized as a disease of 'lifestyle' or 'choice'. This has had clear, and apparently enduring consequences, for the identification of supposedly 'innocent' and 'guilty' victims of the disease. Of particular concern in this respect is the possibility that distinctions such as these may subsequently be used to restrict access to health and social service provision to those who may be popularly perceived as having developed AIDS 'through no fault of their own'.

Given these issues, there is a clear and urgent need for research into the political economy of AIDS. By more clearly identifying the relationship between the economic, political and ideological forces that structure popular and professional responses to AIDS, such work is likely to highlight the strategies of opposition open to those who have been viewed with increasing alarm recent attempts to use AIDS as a means by which to introduce more pervasive and insistent mechanisms of social control. Many social groups have been targetted in this way. They include variously gay men (through demands for compulsory testing and quarantine), young people (through demands for sex education emphasizing abstinence and monogamy), prostitutes (through demands for registration and compulsory testing), black people (through demands for stricter immigration control), injecting drug users (through demands for tougher penalties) and women (through demands that they, rather than their male partners, take the responsibility for safer sex).

At a rather different level, there is also a need to enquire more critically into the nature and consequences of what is popularly termed 'health education' in relation to AIDS. Teachers, educational researchers and those working in advertising have long known that information alone is unlikely to bring about clear-cut changes in behaviour (even if the production of such changes is morally and ethically desirable). The history of public information campaigns relating to tobacco and alcohol consumption in Britain and North America shows that rarely do these these have straightforward cognitive and behavioural consequences (Gatherer *et al*, 1979). Instead, people respond variably to the health education information they receive, and lay beliefs about health and illness have an important role to play in mediating the impact of official health education messages. Too often, it is uncritically assumed that high profile campaigns which use shock and horror to get the message across are all that is required in this respect. Research is urgently needed to identify the forms of health intervention which temper their commitment to the public good with a concern to facilitate individuals in their exploration of a wide range of safer behavioural options.

Given that research into the social aspects of AIDS is still in its infancy, it is not possible to be all embracing in terms of the issues that can be addressed in a book such as this. The picture of social research into AIDS that is painted at any one moment must of necessity be incomplete. Since the authors represented in this book first met, there has been a growth of interest in issues as diverse as women and AIDS, injecting drug use and AIDS, the social phenomenology of AIDS and political intervention around AIDS. These are being explored more fully in a variety of community initiatives and research projects. The outcome of these will be reported on at subsequent conferences concerned with the social and cultural dimensions of HIV infection and AIDS.

References

ALTMAN, D. (1986) *AIDS and the New Puritanism*, London, Pluto Press.
GATHERER, A. *et al* (1979) *Is Health Education Effective?*, London, Health Education Council.

1
Love in a Cold Climate

Jeffrey Weeks

AIDS may be the most serious health crisis to face the world this century. But during its relatively brief history it has become more than a ghastly and relentless disease. It has come to symbolize an age where fear, prejudice and irrationality battle against reason, responsibility and collective endeavour. At the moment it is by no means clear which will triumph.

The reasons for fear are real enough. Some ten million people worldwide may be infected with the HIV virus, the cause of AIDS. Many, perhaps most, of these will go on to get the full blown syndrome. In the USA there have been over 40,000 cases of AIDS, and 20,000 dead. It is estimated that up to two million people carry the virus. AIDS is already the major cause of premature death among adult males in many North American cities. In parts of Central Africa the disease is rife. Estimates vary, but in the next five years we may expect up to one-and-a-half million cases of the illness on the whole continent.

The UK figures are less dramatic but still worrying. There are probably already more than 50,000 HIV carriers. Over 1,000 people at the time of writing have been diagnosed as having AIDS. Half of these are dead. Cases of AIDS are expected to rise six-fold by the end of 1988, to envelop 3000 people. This is a major worldwide health crisis. It has been likened to the great plagues that ravaged Europe in the Middle Ages; and to the influenza epidemic at the end of the First World War which wiped out more people than all the fighting on all the fronts of the war itself.

But this health emergency seems all the more frightening because, at least in the West, we have grown accustomed to the triumphs of medicine in controlling disease. Even with this virus, medical science has shown its efficiency. We now know almost everything there is to know about HIV — *except* how to destroy it. In the meantime, the incidence of AIDS seems to double every ten months.

This was the background to the British government's new sense of urgency at the end of 1986. After months of prevarication — it apparently took a last-ditch direct appeal to the Prime Minister by the permanent Head of the Department of Health and Social Security and the Chief Medical Officer to wrench her into action — the government set up a Cabinet-level committee to coordinate action. An unprecedented health education campaign was launched, with press, radio and TV advertising, a leaflet drop on twenty-three million households, and a £20 million budget. The Health Secretary, Norman Fowler, echoed the words of his advertising copy: 'Stick to one partner; if you don't, use a condom'. And for drug misusers, 'Don't inject drugs; if you can't stop, don't share equipment'.

In the absence for the foreseeable future of a cure or of a vaccine to prevent the spread of the virus, the only safeguard appears to lie with changes in people's behaviour and with the public education to achieve that. This has been clear for some time, and has been the burden of all the expert advice and all the pressure from the groups in the population most affected.

It is some indication of the prejudice and irrationality surrounding the disease that it took so long for the government to adopt a high profile policy on prevention. Here AIDS ceases to be simply a devastating disease and becomes more like a battlefield for conflicting moral and political values, and ways of life.

Popular Responses to AIDS

The popular response to AIDS, the fear and loathing it evokes beyond the actual impact of the disease itself, illuminates a wider crisis of norms and values. Attitudes towards AIDS, and the tardy political reaction, have been shaped by the fact that from its first identification in the USA in 1981 it has been strongly associated with marginalized, oppressed or feared groups; with Haitians, and subsequently with black Americans (a disproportionate number of American sufferers are black); with injecting drug abusers; with prostitutes and with male homosexuals. AIDS has fed easily into wider anxieties and fears that find a focus in powerful streams of racism and homophobia. The result has been predictable and disastrous: a 'moral panic' rooted in a genuine fear of the disease, but seeking scapegoats in those who were the chief sufferers from it.

Moral panics, waves of social anxiety which bring to the surface deep currents of feeling and fear, generally arise in situations of confusion and ambiguity, in periods when the boundaries between legitimate and illegitimate behaviour seem to need redefinition or reclassification. There is a typical stereotyping of the main actors as peculiar types of monsters, leading to an escalating level of fear and perceived threat, the taking up of panic stations and absolutist positions, and a search for symbolic solutions to the dramatized problem.

In the case of AIDS there was a real, anxiety-making disease for which there was no cure, and which seemed to be localized amongst certain groups of people. Irrationally, but predictably, the form the panic took was the search for people to blame. Normally, those suffering from a terrible illness evoke sympathy. Here the victims themselves were stig-matized. Those with AIDS were easily divided into two categories: the 'innocent' (haemophiliacs, female partners of bisexual men, children), and the 'guilty' (drug addicts, the 'promiscuous' and gay men). But it is above all the linkage of AIDS with homosexuality that has dominated attitudes. AIDS is not a specifically homosexual disease, let alone a 'gay plague'. In the Third World it is overwhelmingly a disease amongst heterosexuals. But in most Western countries the main incidence of the illness so far has been amongst gay men. It was only when it began to dawn on people in the last few months of 1986 that AIDS was a general danger that the more vitriolically sensationalist newspapers like *The Sun* — and the government — began to talk of a world health crisis.

The response to AIDS has, however, been more than a moral panic. Trying to understand it is like watching a speeded-up film about the post-war world. Many of the major fears, imagined threats, genuine changes and paranoias pass rapidly before our eyes: the 'break-up' of the family, the presence of 'alien wedges', that elusive phenomenon known as 'permissiveness' ... It is above all changes in sexual mores that have come to symbolize for many people, and especially the moral Right, all the other changes that have taken place. For the former Solicitor General, Sir Ian Percival, the reasons for AIDS were transparent: because 'so many have strayed so far and so often from what we are taught as normal moral behaviour'.[1] And as in many of these debates, it is the 1960s that have become the symbolic focus of these changes.

Charting the New Moralism

There have been three major strands in the moral and sexual shifts of the past generation: a secularization of moral attitudes, a liberalization of popular beliefs and behaviours, and a greater readiness to value and respect social, cultural and sexual diversity. The significance of the AIDS crisis is that it can be used to call into question each of these, and to advance a justification for a return to that 'normal moral behaviour' which acts as a yardstick by which to measure the supposed decline of moral standards.

One of the major changes in the organization of moral behaviour over the past century has been the progressive detachment of sexual norms from religious ones. By the 1960s many of the Christian churches themselves, ranging from the traditionally liberal Quakers to the established Church of England, had effectively abandoned any attempt to impose their own moral values on the whole of society. A distinction was now made between individual morality and social order, with the role of the state being redefined as guaranteeing the latter, not meddling with the former. This was the position broadly endorsed in the great wave of 'permissive legislation' in the 1960s, which reformed the law on homosexuality, abortion, censorship and divorce.

These changes were never accepted by moral conservatives nor by all the churches, and since the 1960s a gathering storm of moral absolutism and 'social purity' has developed. In the US a combination of television evangelism, big money and religious fundamentalism joined hands with new right forces to create the moral majority ('neither moral, nor a majority'). Britain is unlikely to see the emergence of quite such a potent force, but on a range of issues from teenage sex to the representation of sexuality, a moral Right has been mobilized, stretching from the moral rearmament enthusiasms of Mrs. Mary Whitehouse to the post-feminist traditionalism of Victoria Gillick, backed by a chorus of more sinister figures playing their tune in Parliament and elsewhere. [2]

AIDS has proved a golden opportunity for these moral entrepreneurs to raise their profile, to prove to their own satisfaction at least that what they had said all along was right. In recent years there has been growing anxiety about the effects of sexually transmitted diseases such as herpes and hepatitis B. If AIDS is similarly a disease that can be transmitted sexually, then it must prove that 'promiscuity' is not only wrong but, in the inimitable words of a Tory MP, it 'kills'. And gay men, traditionally described as 'promiscuous', and the main victims of the disease in the West, thus become symbolic of the whole moral decline. As Mrs. Whitehouse characteristically put it: 'Over recent years homosexuality has been represented as being perfectly normal ... But now the laughing is over.' [3]

In the age of AIDS, it becomes easier to believe that the limits of medicine and of science have been reached. It therefore makes it potentially more acceptable to seek a moral explanation. 'If AIDS is not an Act of God' thundered the ineffable John Junor in the *Sunday Express*, 'with consequences just as frightful as fire and brimstone, then just what the hell is it?'[4]

This moral revivalism must not be exaggerated. A general liberaliz-ation of attitudes has sunk deep roots since the 1960s, and with it has gone a new willingness to tolerate, if not fully accept, sexual diversity. There has been no major breach in the liberal legal reforms of the 1960s, despite several attempts to restrict access to abortion. Mrs. Gillick's early legal victories in her efforts to prevent doctors providing contraceptive advice to girls under 16 proved pyrrhic. Tory MPs may yet succeed in tightening the laws on obscenity, but despite a huge Conservative majority after 1983 their successes so far have been limited. Even that saloon bar moralist Peter Bruinvels has stated his opposition to attempting to make homosexuality illegal once again.

It is difficult to take Norman Tebbit's attack on the permissive society too seriously when his colleagues are caught dealing with prostitutes and having sex in public lavatories. It seems a little hypocritical to attack one-parent families (which junior minister Rhodes Boyson recently did) when one of your former colleagues notoriously contributed to founding one. It must also be a trifle embarrassing to crusade against drug users when the children of Her Majesty's ministers are amongst them. Senior ministers are products and victims of the major cultural changes of the past generation like everyone else. It does not mean that they will not ride the whirlwind of reaction, but what they can do will be constrained or shaped by the political balance of forces rather than by pure prejudice.

There is considerable evidence that popular attitudes continue to liberalize on many issues, from pre-marital sex to abortion and divorce. There is a greater acceptance of diverse lifestyles and of varied domestic patterns. Even the stigma of illegitimacy is now set for the history books.

There are, nevertheless, significant cross-currents, and homosexuality in particular is caught up in them. Opinion polls suggest that a clear majority of the British public are now against discriminatory laws. But 52 per cent of those interviewed in a recent poll would still prefer not to have a homosexual neighbour, and nearly 70 per cent, according to the *British Social Attitudes* survey, refuse to recognize the legitimacy of lesbian and gay relationships.[5]

Yet, along with the rise of feminism, the emergence of a public lesbian and gay presence has been one of the most dramatic changes in the social and sexual scene over the past thirty years. From being a love that barely whispered its name it has now become highly vocal.

These changes have not gone unnoticed. In the US, mobilization against homosexuality has been a significant element in the New Right's efforts to shape a new majority. Just as feminism can be blamed for profoundly disrupting traditional demarcations between the sexes, homosexuality has been attacked for undermining marriage and the family. Lesbian and gay ways of life are deeply antithetical to the 'pro-family' rhetoric and authoritarian moral values espoused by the New Right.

And the whole issue of the legitimacy of non-traditional sexual relations is a fraught one beyond the bounds of the New Right. Consider for instance the torment and convolutions of the Archbishop of York, Dr. John Habgood, in an interview in the *Daily Mail*. He did not, of course, want to see homosexuals 'beleaguered, threatened and shunned by society'. On the other hand, it was unwise to go to the other extreme. He confessed to regarding homosexuality as a 'misfortune', and he was opposed to seeing homosexuality and heterosexuality as 'two perfectly viable alternatives'.[6]

For the Left, AIDS is an even more difficult topic, cutting across traditional political positions and disrupting other loyalties. The pro-gay policies of the London borough of Haringey, under a radical black leader, have been bitterly opposed both by sections of the white working class and by parts of the black community, because of their supposed threat to the family.

There has been an 'unfinished revolution' in attitudes to sexuality in general and to homosexuality in particular. There have been many fundamental changes in the past thirty years, but their impact has been uneven and fragmented, producing frustration as well as social progress, new tensions as the alleviations of old injustices. Secularization, liberalization, changes in the pattern of relationships have all taken place. But they have left deep residues of anxiety and fear, which AIDS as a social phenomenon has fed on and reaffirmed.

The Challenge of AIDS

AIDS is not a disease of a particular type of person. It has affected, and killed, heterosexuals and homosexuals, women and men, white and black, young and old, rich and poor, the promiscuous and the inexperienced. It is the result not of a way of life but of a virus. Moreover, despite the nature of the illness it causes, HIV is not a particularly strong or infectious virus. This is why AIDS is not transmitted through the air, nor by casual contact, nor by quite intimate activity such as kissing. It is spread only through the exchange of bodily fluids, particularly vaginal fluids, semen and blood.

Some groups of people are currently more at risk than others. But it is misleading to talk about 'risk categories'. This inevitably leads to a confident belief that it is always someone else's disease. The identification of AIDS as a 'gay plague' has potentially disastrous effects. It not only leads to the stigmatization of the disease itself, but it also encourages those who do not see themselves as gay to believe that they will not get it.

It is not high risk 'categories' that spread AIDS, it is high risk activities, those which involve the interchange of bodily fluids. These include genital and anal intercourse without protection, oral sex which involves the swallowing of semen, sexual practices (like fist fucking) which might rupture delicate blood vessels, oral-anal sex, and drug-taking where needles are shared. 'Promiscuity' as such is not the danger. Obviously, the more partners you have the more likely you are to come into contact with someone who is carrying the virus. But it is not the number of partners that constitutes the real danger, it is what you do with them. Nor does drug abuse alone lead to AIDS. It can only do so when blood is exchanged via dirty needles.

Given that at the moment there is no cure for AIDS, and there is unlikely to be one for the next few years, what is clearly essential is that people change their habits sufficiently to avoid high risk activities. Other 'solutions' are clearly impractical or unlikely to work. Injunctions to lifelong monogamy might seem a simple solution, as might giving up drug abuse. But in practice, as the government's advertising effectively concedes, our social natures are a little more recalcitrant than that.

The moral Right has offered more draconian suggestions. These have ranged from the compulsory testing of those at risk, including everyone coming from those parts of Africa where the incidence of AIDS is high, to the segregation of the infected and sick. Leaving aside the racism of these proposals, and the affront to civil liberties they represent, they would demand an unprecented mobilization of resources, and yet would still not stop the virus. Tests are sometimes unreliable; they cannot take account of subsequent infection; and there is virtually no means by which the segregation of huge numbers of people could be effectively policed.

The present Conservative government has not yet ruled out compulsory testing of immigrants, and it is still conceivable that it will make a symbolic gesture along these lines to assuage pressure (opinion polls suggest that there is an overwhelming public demand for compulsory testing of the whole population). But such steps will not stop the spread of HIV infection.

The two practical parts of Health Secretary Norman Fowler's advice to the nation — to use condoms, and avoid sharing needles — are thus not only sensible, they are essential. It has, however, taken a great deal of anguish to reach this stage. When Mrs. Thatcher saw the draft of the first advertising campaign in early 1986 she is reported to have vetoed them with the comment: 'it's like writings on a lavatory wall'. Beyond this are a clear range of anxieties for moral conservatives: would promotion of the use of condoms promote promiscuity? Would mention of anal sex encourage the impressionable to try it? The minutes of Lord Whitelaw's committee which supervized the government's policy will make fascinating reading in thirty years' time.

Even so, certain obvious steps have been baulked at. Advertising has not stressed that free condoms can be obtained for 'family planning' purposes. Despite the support of the health ministers, the government is reluctant to offer free needles to iv drug users from fear that it would be seen to condone drug abuse. Yet something momentous is surely under way. British governments have been traditionally reluctant to intervene too directly in the details of sexual regulation. During the last war millions of condoms were distributed to soldiers as a preventative against VD, but the fiction was allegedly maintained that these were to be used to protect the barrels of guns. Here, for the first time, we see a highly conservative government during its citizens to use protectives, in a massive programme of sex education.

Sex education has been a touchstone issue for the moral Right throughout the West. Publicly provided sex education has been seen as a means for the undermining of parental authority, and as a channel for the promotion of sexual perversion 'on the rates'. As the Thatcher government was contemplating its leap into openness in relation to AIDS, it was also wrestling with attempts by its backbenchers to remove control of sex education from teachers and a growing controversy about the 'positive images' policies of Labour-controlled education authorities. Simultaneously, the Education Secretary, Kenneth Baker, was pandering to pressure from his right-wing by denouncing a gay sex education book for children, *Jenny lives with Eric and Martin*, whose main message seemed to be that gay men could be monogamous too. Yet now we witness the government attempting the biggest, and most radical, sex education programme of all.

It was propelled by the potential enormity of the problem to go further in offering explicit advice than would have seemed conceivable only six months before. It did so because AIDS has ceased to be a minority problem, or a problem of troublesome minorities. It has belatedly been recognized as a problem for the whole of society. The only really important question we need to ask is: how will society cope?

The evidence from the gay community suggests that people can change their habits in response to a perceived danger, and a sense of their responsibilities to themselves and others. The incidence of sexually transmitted diseases has, for instance, dropped significantly — by up to 70 per cent in some London STD clinics — suggesting the impact of a sustained community-based campaign for safer sex.

Many of the support organizations like the Terrence Higgins Trust and Body Positive (for those tested positive for the HIV virus) had their origins in the gay community, and are still to a large extent sustained by it. Clearly, if the public education campaign is to work for the whole population then continuous assistance needs to be provided for help organizations such as these on a major scale. It has been estimated by British Telecom, for instance, that following the inauguration of the government's campaign in November 1986, the Terrence Higgins Trust was receiving 400 phone calls per minute; its resources only allowed it to deal with one.

Voluntary effort, however important, is clearly not enough. The government has bitten the bullet on public education. It still has to confront the resource implications of the fight against AIDS. Labour's spokesman on health matters, Michael Meacher, has estimated that the government needs to spend up to five times the amount allotted by the government.[7] AIDS illustrates above all the need for preventive medicine, for a first-class health service, for collective provision. Yet it has erupted into a political situation where all these have been underfunded or under sustained attack.

There are many other challenges. Insurance companies refuse protection to those they deem to be at risk. People with the HIV virus as well as those with full-blown AIDS are finding themselves discriminated against in jobs and housing. Local neighbourhoods campaign virulently against the establishment of hospices for the dying. Children with AIDS face prejudice at school. Even private hospitals, the darlings of Mrs Thatcher's health policy, refuse to take AIDS patients ... the list is potentially endless.

And looming over all these domestic problems is the possibility of a catastrophe in parts of the Third World, especially Africa, where AIDS is caught up in a cycle of poverty and disease that only a massive redistribution of resources from the North to the South can begin to tackle.

AIDS is much more than a medical problem. It throws a bright search light into the complexities, contradictions, divisions and needs of the modern world. It poses many difficult moral and political challenges. It is still too early to say how these will be met.

On the negative side is the evidence of popular prejudice and government sloth over the past five years. On the positive side is abundant evidence of commitment, courage and responsibility: from the medical profession, from scores of volunteers and from people with HIV infection or with full-blown AIDS themselves. There are two systems of values at play. The future history of the AIDS crisis depends on which of these wins.

Notes

1 See *The Guardian*, 22 November, 1986.
2 See WEEKS, J. (1985) *Sexuality and Its Discontents: Meanings, Myths and Modern Sexualities*, London, Routledge and Kegan Paul, chapter 2.
3 Quoted in *The Guardian*, 22 February, 1985
4 See the *Sunday Express*, 24 February, 1985.
5 See JOWELL, R., WITHERSPOON, S. and BROOK, L. (1986) *British Social Attitudes: The 1986 Report*, Aldershot, Gower.
6 See the *Daily Mail*, 21 November, 1986.
7 See *The Guardian*, 22 November, 1986.

2
Organizing AIDS

Ken Plummer

> Ah, these are desperate times Mrs Lovett, and desperate measures must be taken.
> Stephen Sondheim, *Sweeney Todd*

At the start of the 1980s, 'AIDS' had not been invented. Throughout the previous decade, and maybe earlier, people had been contracting a peculiar *unnamed* disease and sometimes dying from it.[1] The phenomenon of AIDS itself, however, had yet to be perceived. There were no people identified as suffering from it, and the 'AIDS spectrum' — of AIDS and ARC, of PGL and HIV Seropositivity, of the 'worried well' and the 'fear of AIDS' — had not been invented. There were no hospital beds for people with AIDS and no doctors and nurses dedicated to their care. No funds had been directed towards it, no research had been conducted upon it, no blood tests had been organized for it, no government had pronounced around it, no self-help groups had been established to deal with it, no media had talked about it, no moral crusader had campaigned against it, no household had been leafleted about it, no billboard had advertised it and no gay community had been disrupted by it. There were no articles, no journals, no legal handbooks, no nursing guides, no books, no films, no novels, no television programmes, no soap operas, no phone-ins, no videos, no posters, no badges, no pamphlets, no conferences, no concerts, no sick jokes and no obituaries about AIDS. There were no experts on every conceivable aspects of AIDS — no oncologists or virologists, no haematologists or immunologists, no microbiologists or epidemiologists, no venereologists or sociologists, no psychiatrists or psychologists, no health educators or health counsellors, no condom specialists or fund-raisers. AIDS had not entered the discourses of sex and of drugs, of gayness and of prostitution, of race and religion, of haemophilia and blood transfusion, of third world and world health, of therapy and trade unionism, of science and literature, of law and ethics, and of power and control.

Yet now, as I write, AIDS has become all of these things and more. First identified in 1981 and officially named in July 1982, AIDS signposts a syndrome in which the body's immune system is unable to function properly. It is however much more than this, being also a set of powerful — often painful — *social meanings* that emerge through a host of social arenas and are generated in many social practices. AIDS — the biological disease — must therefore be distinguished from 'AIDS' — the social institution.

AIDS is now widely presumed to be a major medical issue, involving the breakdown of the body's immune system and the subsequent invasion of the host by a wide range of opportunist infections and tumours affecting the chest, the gastro-intestinal system, the central nervous system and the skin. It is almost certainly caused by a family of viruses (initially designated HTLV-III, LAV and ARV, and currently known as HIV-I, HIV-II) which are transmitted through bodily fluids and result in a spectrum of diseases. It is pandemic, infectious but not contagious, and its growth rate seems to be near exponential.

By way of contrast, the meanings of AIDS as a social phenomenon are lodged in the institutions and practices of medicine, of self-help, of government and of the media. To take such a view, is to recognize that around an organic disorder has emerged a series of arenas of social action, outside of which AIDS itself cannot exist. Indeed, AIDS as a social entity is organized and constituted through them. Yet it is these profoundly and ubiquitously *social* qualities of AIDS that have so often been ignored. Indeed, a myriad of forces have been required to assemble, manufacture, produce and construct 'the AIDS problem' as we now know it. As Gusfield (1981) has argued,

> Human problems do not spring up full blown and announced into the consciousness of bystanders. Even to recognize a situation as painful requires a system of categorizing and defining events. All situations that are experienced by people as painful do not become matters of public activity and targets for public action. Neither are they given the same meaning at all times by all peoples. 'Objective' conditions are seldom so compelling and so clear in their form that they spontaneously generate a 'true' consciousness. Those committed to one or other solution to a public problem see its genesis in the necessary conditions of events and processes; those in

opposition often point to 'agitators' who impose one or another definition of reality. (p. 3)

To say this is neither to deny the existence of the disease, which would be absurd, not to minimize its impact, which would be inhumane. It is simply to employ an analytic approach which, as Wiener (1981) has remarked in her research into the politics of alcoholism, can show how a:

problem is infused with life: how the dimensions are carved out, how the number of people drawn into concern about these discussions is increased, how a common pool of knowledge begins to develop for the arena participants, and how all these sub-processes increase the visibility of the problem. (p. 14)

But the points I am making here are not merely academic. The social forces which currently 'organize' a problem such as AIDS in certain ways preclude organizing it in others — at least for the time being. In critically examining these constructions, the task is to sense what is *not* being said, who is *not* speaking, where the structured absences lie. It is to ask what themes from the past are being extended through AIDS, and it is to enquire into the way in which the manufacture of the AIDS as a social problem linked to power. While many may disapprove of those who take such a stance, this 'constructionalist' view has the momentary privilege of suspending belief in 'reality'.[2] It allows us to explore in detail the social institutions and practices to which AIDS has given rise. By analyzing events like this, the claims that are made for medical success, the slow advances within technical problem solving and the discovery of new ideas can all for the moment be held in doubt and investigated for their social constitution.

But my task in this chapter is a little more direct than this since it is my intention here to signpost some of the social aspects of AIDS which are amenable to further analysis. A number of these are explored more fully in other chapters in this book. In doing this, I will begin to identify how, in Wiener's (1981) terms, the 'AIDS problem' has been animated, legitimated and demonstrated over the past few years, and now provisional structures, that may form the basis of negotiation and bargaining over the next few decades, have already emerged.

In order to achieve this goal, I will look first at what I will call the *linguistic organization* of AIDS. I will do this by scrutinizing the political languages and rhetorics that have emerged to organize our thinking about the syndrome as a kind of AIDSPEAK. I will focus in particular on the ways in which AIDS has been so quickly medicalized and stigmatized. From this, I will move to consider processes by which AIDS has been *publicly organized* both commercially and in terms of 'moral panic'. Next, I will consider the *personal organization* of AIDS — the processes by which AIDS can be identified, the processes by which people with HIV infection and AIDS come to know themselves and the processes by which the uncertainty associated with the diagnosis of AIDS can be personally managed. Finally, I will look at some of the ways in which AIDS has been *socially* and *culturally organized*. In particular, I will look at the consequences of AIDS for the reorganization of sexuality in general and for gay culture in particular.

Clearly, within this context it would be inappropriate to be other than suggestive in identifying the significant dimensions of these four modes of organisation and in suggesting areas where more research is needed. My task here is merely to begin the task of mapping out the terrain for future research initiatives.

The Linguistic Organization of AIDS: AIDSPEAK

Social life is organized through language, a great deal of which is political (Edelman, 1977). It serves as a cloak which captures minds and organizes the way the world is seen. And since, as Kenneth Burke once remarked, 'every way of seeing is a way of not seeing', it matters hugely what language we use to 'make sense' of AIDS. The power of rhetoric and metaphor in discussing AIDS has long been recognized (Hutton-Williams, 1983) and several chapters in this book address this issue more fully. Whilst the social meanings of AIDS are confused, contradictory and conflictual, here I would like to focus on two obvious, but overpoweringly central, linguistic devices through which our understanding of AIDS has been organized. One of these focusses upon the medicalization of AIDS (and the counter-attack to resist this and demedicalize it), whilst the other focusses upon the stigmatization of AIDS (and the counter-attack to destigmatize it, especially within the gay community). It is hard, and probably impossible in this culture, to think or talk about AIDS without operating within either or both of these rhetorics.

Medicalizing AIDS relies upon the pervasive ideology of the medical model as a way of understanding health and illness. Within this paradigm, the causes of ill-health are located within the body — in the breakdown of tissues and systems — and AIDS itself is conceptualized in an elaborate scientific vocabulary of lymphocytes, antibodies and syndromes. Its specific etiology is said to be lodged in a germ — the Human Immunodeficiency

Virus — and its management lies in hospitalized care and the long-term search for a vaccine.

In sharp contrast, efforts to stigmatize AIDS operate with a set of almost contradictory assumptions. According to this mode of analysis, the problem is located not within the body but in behaviour and lifestyles, and AIDS itself is conceptualized not in scientific terms but morally and theologically via reference to sin, evil and moral irresponsibility. Within this paradigm, AIDS is to be managed not by hospitalization, but by segregation, discrimination and exclusion (Goffman, 1963).

These two ways of thinking about AIDS can be represented as follows (figure 1).

Figure 1: Two dominant rhetorics of 'AIDS'

	Medical Model	**Stigma Model**
Focus	Body/organic	Behaviour/life Style
Mode of conceptualization	Scientific	Moral, political theological
Mode of explanation	Germ-based	Evil, sin, choice, responsibility
Mode of management	Clinical	Segregation, discrimination, exclusion

Of course, these models are overly simple abstractions. Each of them harbours many divergent positions which often come in hybrid form: epidemiology as a mode of analysis, for instance, has its origins in the medical model, but also acknowledges the impact of social factors in the determination of ill health. Similarly, whilst the two models may be mutually exclusive as abstractions, in reality they co-exist in writing about AIDS and in many people's minds. AIDS is therefore lodged within a contradictory discourse. Finally, these two images monopolize nearly all contemporary thinking about AIDS. Although they may be rejected by some, the very act of rejecting them demonstrates their pervasiveness. It is therefore impossible to enter the world of AIDS without entering either the world of medicine or of stigma.

The Medicalization of AIDS and Its Alternatives

The dominance of medical rhetoric is hardly surprising since medicine has become a pervasive social force in western societies. Its application to AIDS therefore seems only logical, sensible and reasonable. So absolutely firm is its grip that it is very hard to imagine AIDS without it. There *is*, after all, a very clear and highly visible organic disability — nothing could be more pronounced than the collapse of the immune system and the subsequent invasion of a person by a host of manifest diseases. There *are* many laboratories dedicated to the scientific exploration of every aspect of the problem. There *is* talk of the 'retrovirus phylogeny' and of 'malignant T-lymphocytes'. There *is* a cluster of highly labile viruses — Human Immunodeficiency Viruses (HIV-I, HIV-II etc) which *can* be viewed microscopically. The disease *is* managed clinically. The search *is* on for a vaccine. Even the very term — Acquired Immune Deficiency Syndrome — has its origins in medical science. Nothing could be clearer and more firmly established. AIDS is medical.

More than this, medicine has made enormous strides in knowledge about AIDS since the syndrome was first identified: viruses have been discovered, a blood test marketed and drugs to control some symptoms found. Claims have been made that, 'At no time in history has so much progress been made on such a complex disease in so short a time' (Brandt, cited in DeVita *et al.*, 1985). AIDS has become in many ways symbolic of medicine's long time claim to be able to 'save the world'. Of course, much of this may be true. But what is odd is the way in which a long tradition which has been subversive of medical thought, a tradition which embraces Montaigne and Molière, Proust and Shaw, and which became particularly prominent during the 1970s, has been significantly ignored in recent discussions about AIDS.

In many ways it is surprising that this medical hegemony should have been so readily embraced over the past five years, because throughout this time and from so many different positions, medicine itself has been under attack. Its achievements have been shown to be less spectacular than many had previously thought, whilst its failures and prejudices have been shown to be manifold. Both from within the medical profession and without, it has been suggested that 'medical intervention has made, and can be expected to make, a relatively small contribution to prevention of sickness and death' (McKeown, 1979). Medicine has been charged with ineffectiveness, and the suggestion has been made that the most significant factors contributing to changes in health may not have been medical, but nutritional and environmental. It has also been argued that the growth of medicine has created a professional dominance which excludes other alternatives (Freidson, 1970); increased social control (Zola, 1972); the generation of exploitative markets and Industrial Medical Empires (Navarro, 1976) and the reproduction of patriarchal relations (Doyal, 1979).

Indeed, it has also been claimed that the 'medical establishment has become a major threat to health'. Far from simply being ineffective or controlling, institutionalized medical practice is actually damaging. In Illich's (1975) classic polemic, *Medical Nemesis/Limits to Medicine* there are three forms this damage can take: clinical (where medical intervention can make the situation worse, even fatally so), social (where the role of medication is extended to a wider and wider range of experience), and cultural (where too much dependency is created and there is a 'paralysis of healthy responses to suffering, impairment and death').

All these arguments have formed the core of a critical medical sociology, in which the benign and progressive interpretations generally attributed to medicine have been subjected to critical evaluation. This is not the place for an extended analysis of such debates, but it is somewhat anomalous that their existence should so far have been largely ignored in discussions of AIDS. It is also all the more surprising then that the gay movement itself should have been relatively mute on such matters, given that in the 1970s it perceived medicine as one of the chief regulators of homosexuality, and spent considerable political effort attacking it. Within less than a decade, the medical profession has moved from being seen as a central oppressor to being seen as a major ally; and, curiously, homosexuality itself has moved from being increasingly demedicalized to finding itself once more entrapped in medical talk (Conrad and Schneider, 1980; Bayer, 1981).

Although there is clearly much of value in medical work, at the very least there should surely be some appraisal of claims such as these and their relevance to contemporary understandings of AIDS. Has AIDS, for example, become a matter of professional dominance — an area of interventional activity in which medicine has established a monopoly on research questions, grants and practices? And does all that is now taken for granted by medicine actually exclude the asking of other questions? There are, for example, a number of rival theories concerning the role of HIV in the etiology of AIDS, but they are hardly ever heard, and medical journals will not publish them.[3] Likewise, has AIDS has been used by the medical profession as a means of extending controls over personal life? Have new exploitative markets been created through the arrival of new drugs and therapies to alleviate some of the symptoms associated with AIDS? Have stereotypes of women and men, and of lesbians and gay men, been reinforced through medical responses to AIDS? Have medical interventions around AIDS actually made the situation worse for many patients? To pose each of these questions is to begin a different way of thinking, one which does not accept the rhetoric of medicine uncritically.

Curiously, the most pervasive challenges that have been made to date on this orthodoxy, however, have come not from critical stances such as these but from the emerging alternative or holistic health movement. The basic ideas have been around for a long time: think positively about life and death; take care of your body through both exercise and diet; try to reduce any stress in your life; and (maybe) take a programme of vitamins. 'Macrobiotics', 'guided imagery', 'acupuncture', 'massage', 'nutrition', 'homeopathy' and 'vitamin C therapy' are prominent as its 'buzz' words (Tatchell, 1986; Van Ness, 1986).

According to this type of analysis, a healthy attitude towards the body and the self may make all the difference between living and dying; between developing AIDS or remaining relatively asymptomatic. Such a point of view argues that since most people with HIV infection do not go on to get AIDS, there must be something other than the virus at work. Likewise, since some 15 per cent of the people diagnosed with AIDS since 1981 are still alive — it is by no means the fatal disease that we are constantly being told it is. Within this alternative rhetoric, it is the attitude of being positive and taking good care of oneself that provides the missing link. At its most extreme — as in some of Spence's (1986) writing, it espouses the view that we are free to choose our own way, and that if we choose the path of life, affirmation and love, all will be well. If only we can develop self-love, eliminate isolation and 'live without limits', then we can transcend the crisis of AIDS and transform it instead into a source of opportunity for self-empowerment. The language used here is distinctly reminiscent of some West Coast self-actualization therapists — 'Listen to your body. It is a mine of information and a masterpiece'. 'Assume your importance in every situation and be seen.' Stay true to the voice within you.' Within this counter-rhetoric (a language which a number of people with AIDS themselves have started to use), there is substantial optimism. In a series of interviews conducted by Nungesser (1986) with people with AIDS, for example, there are many who express such positive attitudes: 'One's attitude is better if one feels and looks better'; 'Be gentle with yourself'.

There are many problems with this alternative way of analyzing things, but most significant is the enormous burden of responsibility which it places back on people who are often very ill. To suggest that people with AIDS are in control of their own destiny is to make them feel guilty if they find they can't control events.

A number of other alternatives to mainstream medical explanation suggest that co-factors may be very much involved in the etiology of AIDS. Many of these suggest that there is some connection between AIDS, stress and lifestyle. There are extreme examples, where all of AIDS is seen as a case of massive collective guilt induced by society's hostility to gays and sex (Schmidt, 1984); and there are also more focussed attempts to establish the role of specific co-factors. *Death Rush*, for instance, is a sharply written North American book by two gay activists who argue that the virus in itself is not sufficient cause of AIDS; poppers and other drugs are much more crucial. Their advice is blunt: 'Don't use poppers. This is the first and last thing to be said about them' (Lauritsen and Wilson, 1986). This book enters the arena of medical science by providing a long medical bibliography of evidence which supports their thesis that toxic, recreational drugs of all kinds (including alcohol, but especially the nitrite inhalants) are key co-factors in causing immune breakdown. Yet the authors are not medics, but gay activists, and their model is not simply medical (or toxicological, in their case) but moral. Their aim is clearly to change existing patterns of behaviour. Here, as everywhere, the practical divide between the rhetoric of medicine and the rhetoric of morality is very hard to define (Kingham, 1987).

The Stigmatization of AIDS and Its Alternatives

If one of the major languages in which AIDS has been organized is medical, then the other has been that of stigma. Without doubt, AIDS as a disease has been mapped on to intense devaluation, discreditability, dishonour and degradation. Many diseases — like leprosy and tuberculosis — have held this potential in the past, and some — like cancer or epilepsy — still hold it today (Sontag, 1983). But in the contemporary world, AIDS has almost become synonymous with the most profound stigma — a connection which it seems almost impossible to avoid. Even though media workers and educationalists, lay people and gay people may try to resist it, somehow this has become the omnipresent fact of AIDS. Some cultures have even tried to deny the existence of AIDS altogether — so deep lies the stigma. And as anyone who has found themselves placed somewhere on the AIDS spectrum (as HIV antibody positive, as having ARC or even as being 'at risk') knows, to be diagnosed thus is to be forced to confront (and hopefully resist) deep discreditability. In this respect, it has recently been suggested that AIDS is an illness with a triple stigma: it is connected to stigmatized groups, it is sexually transmitted and it is a terminal disease. In fact, AIDS is much more than this because its connections to stigma are multiple.

The stigma of AIDS is derived from many sources. In the oldest meanings of the word, there are, for some, actual *physical bodily* marks that serve as stigmata. The blotches that signpost the presence of Kaposi's sarcoma and the physical disabilities that some people with AIDS experience — extreme loss of weight, skin disease, lymphadenopathy, mobility problems — all link them to the stigma that has traditionally been the lot of the disabled. Peabody (1986) in a powerful autobiography of a mother caring for a dying son, describes the stigmatized look thus:

> the body itself is gaunt, knobby, emaciated, and it hunches over and shuffles along, weak with malnourishment. And the face — the face is prematurely aged. Men of 30 appear years older, the skin stretched tight over cheek and jawbones, wrinkling dryly and painfully when they smile. The hair is thin and has lost its sheen. The eyes are torturous, sunk deep into their bone-ridged hollows, the eyelashes and brows sparse, and their spareseness accentuating the eyes, giving faint parenthesis to the message, 'Why me?' — and to the eternal plea for help, for life. And though they hate to be called it, they are victims. Not of their chosen lifestyle, but of society's prejudice, its unwillingness to help them, to answer their plea. My son has an AIDS face. (p. 154)

But the stigma goes much deeper than this by connecting to the inner blotches as well: the stigmas of moral character. For the language of AIDS is firmly grounded in two of the deepest, longest surviving structures of stigma: erotophobia and racism. To these may be added other long held fears — notably of drugs and death. AIDS contains a striking mapping together of many elements of fear in the social psyche. Of course, this is too big a generalization to make. If AIDS is now a world phenomenon, these same fears are almost certainly not universal, world-wide ones. AIDS will offer a unique opportunity to see which cultures provide the less stigmatizing responses.

Within the context of this chapter, there is no space to analyze all these stigmatizing messages. Nevertheless, probably the most commonly encountered stories about AIDS are those which link it directly to 'promiscuous homosexuality', 'prostitution', 'casual sex', and 'drug abuse'. Of course, each of these practices has its own history of stigmatization which antedates AIDS by many years. But each has also found itself the focus of heightening hysteria since AIDS in the form of new 'moral purity' campaigns, new drug campaigns and new attacks on homosexuality (Vass, 1986).

In December 1986 at a conference on AIDS, James Anderton — Chief Constable of Greater Manchester and President of the Association of

Chief Police Officers — bluntly captured the core of this idea when he said, 'Everywhere I go I see increasing evidence of people swirling around in a human cess-pit of their own making'. AIDS is a 'self-inflicted scourge' (*The Guardian*, 1986).

But it is homosexuality that has been most centrally attached to AIDS — at least in the western world. This is not surprising: early medical work was instrumental in welding them together when it originally called the syndrome GRID — Gay Related Immune Disease, and indeed the categories which are used to collect official statistics still do. The mass media too was quick to coin terms like the 'gay plague' and the 'gay bug', and although this has now generally ceased, images of 'innocent' and 'guilty' victims are still pervasive. Even the gay community has long had a curious ambivalence about AIDS — on the one hand trying to deny the intimate connections between gayness and AIDS, and on the other simultaneously reorganizing nearly all its energies and activities towards the syndrome — from fund-raising and political debate to a massive proliferation of self-help groups. Much of this, of course, has served to heighten the connection between AIDS and homosexuality in the public eye. Yet the link between AIDS and homosexuality is misconceived. Many people with AIDS are neither homosexual nor bisexual; the lesbian experience, for example, is that least likely to be engulfed by the disease. Homosexualities are as varied experiences as heterosexualities and harbour many diverse forms, some of which can in no way be connected to AIDS. Further, although initial reports on the origins of AIDS concerned white middle class gay men in New York and San Francisco, subsequent analysis has suggested that the genesis of AIDS was outside of gay circles. Yet for many, AIDS and homosexuality have been merged — giving to AIDS its key stigma whilst heightening the stigma that already existed of being gay.

Racism is another deep structure onto which the fear of AIDS has been mapped. The major rival explanation for the origins of AIDS to that of homosexuality have connected it to 'blacks'. In the earliest reports, Haitians were identified as a 'high risk' group and extreme stories about blood drinking and voodoo rites began to circulate (Moore and Le Barou, 1986). When these subsided, and the Centers for Disease Control in Atlanta, Georgia stopped calling Haitians a 'high risk' group, the emphasis shifted to Africans, and the suggestion was made that the genesis of AIDS lay on that continent. A whole new 'fear of foreigners' subsequently developed, and many countries are now testing — and even expelling — black visitors from Africa.[4] But this general connection conceals a deeper problem.

In North America some 25 per cent of all persons with AIDS are black (overall, black people make up only 12 per cent of the US population), and in some cities like New York the figure is much higher. Yet very little is being done to meet the AIDS-related needs of black communities in the US — where homophobia is expressed very differently and where 'coming out' may be more difficult; where drug use may be more common and where imprisonment is more frequent. Within such communities, there is a pressing need also for steps to be taken to meet the needs of women and children with AIDS. Yet, whilst the general stigma linking AIDS to black people continues, the concrete needs of black people in this respect continue to go ignored.

The Public Organization of AIDS — AIDSPANIC

AIDS has become *the* disease of the late twentieth century. In everyday life, from media-watching to pub talk, AIDS is rarely out of public consciousness. In scientific circles, thousands of delegates with hundreds of papers jet around the world for international symposia. Research bibliographies abound, and by 1987 there were already at least nine journals dedicated to writing on AIDS.[5] All governments have had to take notice of the epidemic: more than 200 bills have been introduced in state legislation across North America in 1986 alone. In November 1986, the UK government finally established its own AIDS Committee under Lord Whitelaw and announced a £20 million public information campaign which would leaflet every household in the land — a quite unprecedented act. The World Health Organization has announced that AIDS is its major priority, and an enormous AIDS industry — medical, moral and media — has been built up around the syndrome. AIDS has become both omnipresent and omnipotent. It is the disease — but also the symbol — of our age.

Superficially, so much fuss is surprising. Though every case is a profound tragedy, by January 1987 there were still only around 700 people with AIDS in the United Kingdom. Thus, when compared with other diseases, the mortality rate is still very low. Assuming that the five-year toll from 1982 to 1986 of deaths related to AIDS in the UK was about 350, then in just one of these years (1985) there were some 134,000 deaths from cancer, 190,000 deaths from heart disease and 5000 deaths from road accidents. Many other distressing diseases — cervical cancer, Alzheimer's disease, 'cot deaths', sickle cell anaemia (all of which have heavy tolls and costs) — have received correspondingly little attention. Why haven't these been so widely reported and discussed? What factors have led to this enormous and unprecedented interest in AIDS?

There are, in fact, many good reasons for this concern. It is not the absolute numbers now, but their future projections, that matters. Although making predictions of this sort is an extremely hazardous task, and one which is prone to errors of all sorts (points taken up in Coxon's contribution to this book), cautious projections for the UK made in late 1986 suggested some 2000 cases of AIDS by 1988. Less cautious estimates suggested that there might be 10,000 cases by the year 1990. When we take into account not just AIDS itself but the full spectrum of AIDS-related disease, then estimates escalate (to around 300,000 affected people in the UK by the year 1990; Wells, 1986). When the world pandemic is considered, the figures can become alarming. In the US alone, there have already been well over 30,000 diagnosed cases of AIDS (57 per cent of whom are dead) and in Central Africa, there are an estimated five million people with AIDS (Sabatier, 1986). When we add to this the disturbing characteristics of AIDS, it is not hard to see why there has been so much concern. AIDS is a dreadfully painful syndrome which opens up the body to a wide spectrum of agonizing diseases — debilitating diarrhoea, brain disorders and seizures, pneumonias and cancers, internal cripplings which make movement difficult and which result in wasting away. As a syndrome AIDS is probably unique in causing so much death and so much suffering amongst such a relatively young age group. In the US, 22 per cent of people with AIDS are in their twenties, 47 per cent are in their thirties and another 22 per cent are in their forties (Devita *et al.*, 1985). All of this is sufficient to justify the enormous interest in AIDS. Human concern is 'naturally' aroused when the magnitude of suffering is so great.

But all is not quite so benign as this analysis might suggest. Although AIDS has undoubtedly brought forth the positive face of human concern, it has a darker side. For AIDS has become a symbol for advancing the interests and powers of many groups; and it has fuelled many major social anxieties.

Thus, religious groups such as the Moral Majority in North America have been able to present AIDS as a evidence of 'God's revenge' on permissiveness: 'There'd be no AIDS epidemic in the West if the laws of Moses had been followed'. Moral campaigns such as these have a long history, but in recent months they have been quick to coopt AIDS as a means to achieving their ends (Brandt, 1985).

Medical groups too have not only found in AIDS an intriguing scientific problem that straddles many disciplines, but also an area of research where grants can be readily attained and careers established. The road to the Nobel Prize is paved with AIDS research. Even within the gay community itself — devastated as it has been by AIDS — new career opportunities and funding has been created around AIDS. Perhaps most important of all, the mass media, in all its forms, has found that AIDS sells. Elsewhere in this book, reference is made to the massive and stigmatizing media coverage there has been of AIDS (Vass, 1986; Feldman and Johnson, 1986).

In a process akin to a cybernetic 'feed-back loop', a small system rapidly expands to take on a life of its own. An enormous network of AIDS-oriented groups now exist on an international scale and is likely to grow. Each is establishing its own bureaucracy and mode of organization; its own personnel and ideology; its own sources of funding; its own career structures and resources. Organizations emerging now in the mid-1980s are likely to carve out and shape the problem for the future. AIDS has indeed become an industry.

But apart from these self-generating organizations and interests, there are deeper reasons for concern about AIDS, ones that have their roots in both history and the contemporary human psyche. At the most obvious level, AIDS has become a massive scapegoating device, neatly dividing the world into the 'guilty' and the 'innocent' by selectively blaming some of its 'victims'. But as Weeks so astutely remarks elsewhere in this book, AIDS is more than a simple moral panic in which convenient scapegoats have to be found for modern social anxieties. Rather,

> It is like watching a speeded up film about the post-war period. Many of the major fears, imagined threats, genuine changes amid paranoias pass rapidly before our eyes: the 'break up' of the family, the presence of 'alien wedges', that elusive phenomenon known as 'permissiveness' ... It is above all changes in sexual morals that have come to symbolize for many people and especially the moral right, all the other changes that have taken place.

Scapegoating needs fears to feed on, and free-floating fears of 'permissiveness' have become abundant around AIDS, generating a whole gallery of monsters. There is, however, nothing new about this scapegoating of those who are the 'victims' of disease; the Black Death scapegoated the Jews and massacred them, the plagues scapegoated sinners, cholera was against the great unwashed, syphilis rooted out whores. Disease and moral scapegoating have long historical connections (Porter, 1986).

But there are even wider anxieties than these involved in AIDSPANIC. For one thing, AIDS puts at risk the common belief in medical progress. Most people in the Western world have come to assume that plagues are a thing of the past, having been 'conquered' by modern medicine. Nowadays, degenerative diseases have come to replace many of the old contagions as the major threats to health and well being. Yet this, of course, is only partially true. There have been, and there continue to be, regular outbreaks of contagious disease in this century: from the great wave of influenza which emerged towards the end of the First World War, killing 'twenty million or more' (McNeill, 1979) to the sleeping sickness which emerged in Austria in 1917 and was subsequently transmitted to some five million people in the Western world (about a third of them dying in the acute stage); from the US polio epidemic of 1916 in which some 6000 people died, to the much smaller epidemic of Legionnaires Disease amongst some 200 people staying at a Philadelphia hotel in 1976. But all these are small compared with the great ravages of the past: leprosy, plague, smallpox, syphilis, scarlet fevers and tuberculosis. In a prophetic and ominous observation, DuBos (1959) remarked:

> In Europe, leprosy was prevalent in the fourteenth century, plague in the fifteenth, smallpox in the seventeenth and eighteenth centuries, scarlet fever, measles and tuberculosis in the nineteenth century and tuberculosis in the twentieth century. No one was prepared for the fury of the influenza epidemic when it struck after World War 1. Who can say what is in store for the future and how effective the modern methods of prophylaxis and treatment, the vaccines and drugs, would have proved in the face of these killing epidemics to which Western man had not developed any natural resistance at the time they reached him. (p. 190)

Who can say indeed? Our growing awareness of the fallibility of medicine is also linked to a growing awareness of our own mortality and death.

For many social theorists, death has become the omnipresent symbol of our time; and to the images of Auschwitz, Hiroshima and Vietnam, AIDS may shortly be added. These theorists, however, often overstate the symbolic power of death, since most cultures in the past have had to live with the knowledge of plague, pestilence, poverty and famine (and indeed still do today in the non-Western world).

But there is something more final and more of human creation in contemporary symbolism. Lifton's (1976 and 1979) psychohistorical research has possibly the greatest relevance here, although he has not yet addressed the subject of AIDS itself.[6] In a series of studies, he has spoken with the 'survivors' of extreme situations in which people were immersed in death; of the 'life in death' in Hiroshima and in those 'home from the war' in Vietnam. Out of such research he has generated an understanding of modern life as being based on a 'new wave of millenial imagery — of killing, dying and destroying on a scale so great as to end the human narrative'. His prime concern now is with 'nuclearism' and the 'nuclear image', but he goes further than this to 'explore the psychological relationship between the phenomenon of death and the flow of life'. Moving away from Freud's depth erotic concerns, Lifton sees the contemporary crisis as one of symbol formation — of constructing symbols which allow us a 'sense of continuity (or symbolization of immortality)' when death and dislocation abounds. There are many problems of course with Lifton's work, but there is much in it that may be valuable for future thought about AIDS. It opens the spectre of wide-ranging and free-floating social anxiety around death, immortality and survival. AIDS has been linked, overwhelmingly, with death — even though in reality people with AIDS die at different rates and some 'survive' for many years.

But this death symbolism links to much wider social anxieties. Feeding as it so easily does into status and material interests, AIDS connects to a wider morality play of desire, drugs and deviance. It taps into our interest in medicine and ultimate death. These concerns, however, are not simply grounded in the disease itself, but also in what it stands for — its potent symbolism.

The Personal Organization of AIDS: Identifying and Managing Aids

Not only has AIDS to be recognized publicly before it can become a 'social problem', it also has to be recognized personally before it can become an *illness*. As Locker (1981) has remarked:

> Diseases and illness are then distinct phenomena. Disease is a category applied to a variety of biological events such as changes in physiological, biochemical or anatomical structure and functioning. As biophysical states these events exist independently of human knowledge and evaluation. By contrast, illness is a social state created by human evaluation; it is a symbolic ordering of affairs by the application of a label. Consequently, it is not an entity but a meaning used to explain, organize and evaluate these events or states of affairs. (p. 4)

The processes by which health workers and their patients come to interpret bodily signs as symptomatic of patterns of illness and produce regimes for 'coping' with this have long been of interest to medical sociologists. There is, already, a substantial research literature relating to these concerns which provides paradigms for future enquiry (see, for example, Suchman, 1965;

Fabrega and Manning, 1972; Dingwall, 1976; Kotarba, 1983; Strauss, 1975; Tuckett, 1976; Wortman and Dunkel-Schetter, 1979).

In one sense AIDS is a fairly easy disease syndrome to identify and manage. Its most pronounced symptomatic disorders — chronic diarrhoea, 'wasting', Kaposi's sarcoma, pneumonia — along with the presence of HIV infection itself, would seem to make its recognition a straightforward matter of medical expertise. Medical texts abound with lists of markers and identifying opportunistic diseases, and certainly in its more advanced stages, it must be difficult not to be aware of it. Likewise, most of the opportunistic diseases associated with AIDS are well-known and hospitals have long had to manage the care of those affected by them. Or so it would seem.

In fact, AIDS is a 'diverse disease' and its successful transformation into an illness is a complex process which involves sophisticated social negotiations by a variety of parties (Patton, 1985). Liberace could go to his tragic grave not knowing — or believing nobody else knew — that he 'had AIDS', and only his celebrity status forced the post-mortem diagnosis into the open. How many others have thus kept AIDS as an illness at bay?

Given the complexities associated with defining AIDS, the multiplicity of diseases linked to it, the wide array of symptoms generated by it, the massive variability in the pace of its progress and the stigma and secrecy that engulf it, recognizing AIDS itself can be no easy matter. Worse, AIDS is only the iceberg tip of a vast spectrum of new and hidden disorders — the AIDS spectrum (figure 2).

This spectrum has been progressively extended as more and more linked disorders have been found, but the lines between them are not clear and the pathways from being seropositive to having full-blown AIDS are complex and as yet unknown.

All of this means that identifying AIDS is not really a straightforward matter. At the very least, this raises doubts about the validity of some of the AIDS statistics frequently cited. In this respect, there is a whole political epidemiology of AIDS to be researched. This will involve looking at the political origins and functions of seemingly neutral statistics. For example, sociologists have long recognized that official statistics do not measure some unproblematic reality 'out there'. Instead, official statistics are the product of a series of complex social processes — recording skills, reportability, and wider pressures like media, community and government concern. Statistics can be widely transformed through changes in the processes which define them. How then does one particular experience become an AIDS statistic and another not? How might one agency's system of recording and decision-making differ from that of another? In

Figure 2: *The spectrum of HIV infection*

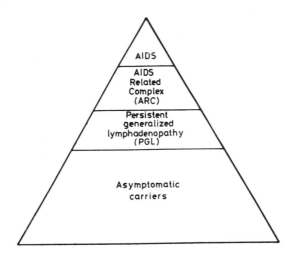

Source: Daniels (1985)

San Francisco or New York, London or Paris, there may be better organized systems for recording, since the numbers being dealt with are relatively large. Indeed the 'efficiency' of these counting processes may actually inflate the recorded numbers of cases because of researchers' concern not to miss a single case of AIDS; an epidemiological self-fulfilling prophesy may thereby take place. But in smaller towns and cities, systems of recording may be less attuned to detecting the presence of AIDS. Furthermore, in some African countries, the problem of gaining accurate estimates of disease prevalence are notorious.

This is certainly not to dismiss statistics out of hand, but to suggest the need for caution in their interpretation. National rates, for example, may conceal many subtle local variations. In San Francisco, for example, 89 per cent of people with AIDS are gay, but in Bel Glade, Florida, people with AIDS are overwhelmingly heterosexual. In New York, drugs and race loom large and in Edinburgh the rate of HIV infection is said to be 60 per cent amongst some injecting drug users. Likewise, a number of broad statistical generalizations that are commonly made about AIDS need to be treated with caution. For instance, the claims have often been made that the number of people with AIDS doubles every six months; but this is not true now in general, and never has been in many more specific contexts. Similarly, it has sometimes been suggested that 5 per cent or even 20 per cent of people infected by HIV will subsequently develop AIDS; but given our present understanding of the epidemic, it is far too early to make such estimates. Finally, it has been argued that one million, one-and-a-half million, two million people or maybe even four million people in the US are seropositive for HIV; but what do such widely varying estimates really mean?

Statistics like these may currently have little reliability or validity, and the authors who originally cite them are frequently cautious in the claims they make. But they are often taken out of context by the mass media and thereby become one more part of public rhetoric about AIDS. Used in this way, they may help substantiate a largely fictional world.

Becoming a Person on the AIDS Spectrum

Of all the processes involved in identifying AIDS, the most central is the way in which people on the AIDS spectrum come to identify and make sense of their illness: how they move from a situation where 'nothing unusual is happening' through some 'problematic experience' where cues from the body are taken to indicate 'trouble' to the decision to seek (or not to seek) medical advice; how they handle the initial diagnosis; how they may enter or resist a sick role; how they may embark upon an illness career, develop lay theories about the disease and establish coping strategies for dealing with emerging problems. Sociologists have studied these social processes for several diseases, but with respect to AIDS research in this field is as yet underdeveloped. What exists at present are psychosocial models of adaptation (Coates *et al.*, 1984; Forstein, 1984; Miller and Green, 1985; Morin *et al.*, 1984; Nichols, 1985) and first hand accounts of what it is like to experience AIDS (Nungesser, 1986). Nearly all of this work has focussed on the experiences of gay men, and the processes by which people cope with AIDS may differ significantly depending on whether the origins of the syndrome are paediatric, drug-related, haemophilia-related or African. Furthermore, as time moves on it may become apparent that the meanings which surround the initial diagnosis of AIDS shift too.

Some researchers have claimed to identify various stages of response to a diagnosis of AIDS similar to Kubler-Ross's (1970) stages of dying. Thus Forstein (1984) has suggested that the person with AIDS is likely to pass through four stages: an initial one of 'shock numbness and disbelief'; followed by 'denial', 'bargaining' (why me?), and 'planning realistically for death'. Nichols (1985) has suggested that situational stress around AIDS may move through three key phases: the inital 'crisis' phase — of 'denial alternating with periods of intense anxiety'; a transitional stage 'when alternating waves of anger, guilt, self pity and anxiety supercede denial'; and a 'deficiency state' of acceptance, where a new stable identity is formed and a more positive lifestyle comes to be built around AIDS.

Stage models like these can be useful analytic tools, but they are all guilty of attempting to impose too much order on actual inchoate experience. Miller and Green (1985), for example, have remarked with respect to stage models such as that of Kubler-Ross that, 'The picture seen by us in patients with AIDS has, however, been much more variable. There is no sign that all patients with AIDS necessarily pass through all these stages'. These comments suggest that it may be more useful to make sense of the events that follow medical diagnosis by identifying recurrent themes. Two of these seem worthy of detailed attention — *anxiety* and *uncertainty*.

Earlier, distinctions were made between AIDS itself (sometimes known as full-blown AIDS) and the illnesses which characterize the rest of the AIDS spectrum. Whilst there has been much public debate about the former of these diagnostic categories, relatively little has been said about the latter. Yet it is here, in the grey area that *could* pre-figure AIDS, that uncertainty is maximized, and support is likely in some ways to be most needed. To be diagnosed as HIV antibody positive or to have the signs of symptoms of either PGL or ARC is to encounter the fears and expectations of full-blown AIDS itself. As one person in this situation said,

> I don't know how to live my life anymore in the basic ways. If I'm going to get AIDS and die within a couple of years, then I'd rather not continue with school. I'd want to use the time differently ... I don't even know if it's all right to kiss my lover anymore. Maybe the worst part of this is just not knowing. (Morin *et al.*, 1984)

Uncertainty then is a pervasive state of being associated with the AIDS spectrum: uncertainty over the nature of the disease, uncertainty over its possible trajectory; uncertainty about the reactions of others, including close friends, family and lovers.

A second closely related theme is that of anxiety. All groups of people on the AIDS spectrum are likely to experience this, but one particular group deserves special mention: the 'worried well', that group in the population which will surely grow larger who are worried about developing AIDS but who are well, in that they show no objective signs of AIDS-related illness. Closely allied to this group, yet different from it, are those who develop 'pseudo-AIDS', where the fear of infection generates the anxiety symptoms which mimic the prodromal features of AIDS itself — sweating, lethargy, rashes, appetite and weight loss (Miller *et al.*, 1985). Here we can find evidence of the medical self-fulfilling prophesy, where the identification of a disease can actually generate some of its symptoms in those who are otherwise well.

The Social Organization of AIDS: AIDS-Impact

That AIDS is having an enormous impact and will continue to do so well into the next millenium is beyond dispute. The numbers, the growth, the age distribution, the toll of pain, the dependency, the death — all will have an unmistakable impact on societies all over the world. In economic terms, the cost of AIDS in terms of new resource needs and lost labour could be devastating (Wells, 1986). In psychological terms, the levels of grief and mourning may even come to surpass the combined effects of holocausts and world wars together.

Yet beyond the pains and cost of the disease itself are the social meanings of AIDS, spreading out everywhere to refashion whole aspects of society. At the core of all this is the person with AIDS. To know you have AIDS is to be constantly aware that you have more than just a disease, it is to embark upon a profound symbolic reordering of your life.

With AIDS there can be no missing the central impact of the breakdown of the immune system which opens up enormous disease possibilities as well as the possibility that one might actually lose one's mind. People become 'so weak, so wasted' (Nungesser, 1986). These problems are *intrinsic* to AIDS. Nobody can deny their impact. But side by side are the *extrinsic* problems of AIDS — those which are not harboured in the disease itself, but which have their origins in the social meanings surrounding it. Of course, such a distinction is only analytic. In practice, meanings and bodies intermingle. Nevertheless, it is helpful to recognize that the person with AIDS confronts not only bodily diseases but also potential guilt, potential stigma, potential secrecy, potential self-blame, potential dependence on medicine and potential awareness of imminent death. Even the meanings of pain associated with the immune breakdown have to be interpreted, and this can only be done through the repertoire of available symbols (Kotarba, 1983).

Imagine what AIDS could be like if the meanings surrounding it were more positive. If there was no stigma attached, if it wasn't termed a 'killer disease', if it wasn't a 'gay plague', if it wasn't 'caused by sexual promiscuity'. There are signs that when the deep stigmas and medical meanings are removed, the illness manifests itself in less severe forms (Tatchell, 1986). The sufferings of people with AIDS are compounded by symbols. And from them the suffering spreads out in ripples — through all

those on the AIDS spectrum and their loved ones, friends and families —
into the wider communities.

The Reorganization of Gay Culture

In the Western world, it is within the gay community that the most
dramatic impact of AIDS has been experienced. Modern gay culture dates
back to the nineteenth century but has constantly been subject to change
as the wider culture has responded to it. In the 1970s, after the 'Stonewall
Riots' occurred in New York City, a new 'liberation' culture and politics
emerged which sought to positively transform gay identities.[8] Now,
however, there are efforts to do this once more. For AIDS has become the
key to a new gay consciousness. Especially in cities with large gay
populations — New York, Los Angeles and San Francisco in the US,
Berlin, Paris, Amsterdam and London in Europe — it is hard to find a gay
man who has not been affected by AIDS in some way or another. Indeed,
whereas in the 1970s, the key to understanding gay life lay in the
politicization flowing from 'Stonewall' and the Gay Liberation Front, now
it has become AIDS that shapes the gay community. As one gay man has
put it, 'There's a whole new batch of gay men in the mid-twenties and
younger who see the health crisis, *not* Stonewall, as the decisive historical
force shaping their gay identity'. Or, as another anonymous gay man has
put it, 'AIDS has infected my dreams'.

AIDS has had a dual impact on the gay community — simultaneously
decimating it and, ironically, strengthening it. The impact has not been
the same everywhere — Nottingham is not New York. At its worst, gay
men have likened the arrival of AIDS to the holocaust. Some have found
whole friendship networks killed off and gay culture has been infused with
an awareness of death and dying that is probably unique in modern
history. Even as early as 1982, one gay commentator could say that he had
already lost thirty of his friends; and one New Yorker, asked in 1984 how
many people he knew with AIDS, could reply: 'about nine hundred'
(Nungesser, 1986). It is not just the death of your lover, or the death of
your best friends who you have nursed for several years, or the death of the
many faces you used to know across a crowded bar, or even the profound
awareness of your own potential mortality that matters. It is the sum total
of all this grief; an enormous psychological crippling that must be added
to actual death.

And yet, out of all this suffering, gay men have organized themselves
into a new culture of resistance: they have fought back through a whole

arena of new organizations. The old gay movement hardly survives: what has taken its place is a massive proliferation of self-help groups covering every aspect of the health crisis.

In New York City, Gay Men's Health Crisis (GMHC) was formed early in 1982, and has grown to handle every aspect of the problem — from public education to sponsoring medical research, from a hot-line that handles over 2000 calls a week to the provision of clinical services for fifty to sixty new cases of AIDS each month; from the 'buddy system' where 'buddies' work on the simple chores that people with AIDS cannot manage, to advocates for legal and financial problems; from a network of support for partners, parents, women and the bereaved, to care for non-gay populations who have been much less capable of significant organization. GMHC is only one of many such organizations around the world — each with their own organizational structure that would rival any corporation, funding which in some cases runs into millions of dollars, and the ability to employ many staff. In England too, the Terrence Higgins Trust has grown from very small beginnings to become a large agency playing a strategic role. Gay leaders have moved from an anarchistic revolutionary politics in the 1970s to a professionalized, bureaucratized politics in the 1980s (Plummer, 1985a, 1985b and 1986).

Reorganizing Sexuality

Since the late 1960s, some sociologists have been keen to argue that human sexuality is *not* an 'imperious, insistent and often impious force that presses universally for release and satisfaction from within the human body' (Plummer, 1982). It is *not* an inevitable biological given, but an experience which emerges through its social environment: it is socially constructed, symbolic and densely scripted. Sexual meanings can be dramatically transformed across cultures, groups and even individuals. This is not the place to elaborate upon this 'constructionist' view of sexuality; but it does have strong implications for understanding sexuality in the age of AIDS (Gagnon and Simon, 1973; Simon and Gagnon, 1986).

The 1960s and 1970s were a period in which sexual meanings were significantly reorganized in pockets of the Western world. With profound changes in demographic structure, family organization, media, economy, polity and urban structures all taking place, it was a period when new sexual identities could become solidified, new sexual institutions could emerge, sex could be used for different social purposes, and shifts in sexual meanings became manifest. Two areas where this was most visible were those of feminist politics, which reconstructed female desire and even feminized sexuality (Snitow, 1986; Vance, 1984; Ehrenreich, 1986), and gay politics, which refashioned conceptions of the erotic. It is the latter which I will be most concerned with here.

For some gay men not only developed a new sense of identity, many actively constructed new scenes and scripts for organizing sexual eroticism — from disco eroticism, the clone culture, the backrooms, the porn stores through to the sado-masochistic bathhouses of pure lust. None of this was wholly new, but the extent of its organization and public accessibility to men was. And with this came new debates — around sadomasochism, paedophilia, fist fucking, poppers; and political claims that linked male gay liberation to the gay male celebration of sex, to the radical claims that gay sex was 'sex incarnate'. Human sexual meanings were literally reconstructed during the 1970s by some gay men (White, 1980; Bronski, 1984; Weeks, 1985; Altman, 1986).

But if sexualities can be transformed in one period then they can be transformed again in another. I do not wish to suggest that such changes can ever be easy, because sexual cultures have histories, structures, institutions and ideologies which give them a semi-permanence; people become committed to their particular forms of sexuality; and there is usually resistance in both culture and personal life to change. But change is nevertheless omnipresent.

The arrival of AIDS had sent shivers out into the gay world by 1982; and at the time of writing, it is doubtful that many gay men in city communities could not have heard of AIDS. Again, I do not simply mean the disease *per se* — the biological world where viruses may be transmitted through semen and lead to immune breakdown. I mean the symbolic meaning of AIDS which basically brings the dreadful message heard through generations of Western culture that sex is a danger: Stop! The reorganization of sex into pleasure, diversity and celebration which was one message of the 1960s and 1970s is ceasing and the old stigmas have re-emerged. From its earliest notification, AIDS has had the potential to be grafted on to the deep structures of sexual hatred. Fragments of the gay movement identified this immediately, and by early 1982 had already made distinctions between high and low risk sex. Debates on sexuality have proliferated in the gay community since then, and have pre-figured issues that only now in 1987 are entering other worlds — especially heterosexual ones. With a curious irony, contemporary gay discourses may actually be shaping the wider sexual discourses of the twenty-first century.

Again, the full complexity of these debates cannot be analyzed yet; but three particular stances can be briefly mentioned: the 'traditionalists', the 'safer sexers' and the 'fuckers'. 'Traditionalists' want a return to what they see as the long established values of monogamy and celibacy. Within the gay world, some argue that the life style of the 1970s which centred on 'fast lane sex' was indeed damaging; and the way forward should be on effectively abandoning sex. Monogamous loving relationships are the blueprint for the future. And since the incubation period of the virus is long, celibacy and chastity are to be preferred. In this view, we are entering the post sexual era; and at its more extreme edge it is leading to the battle on sexual compulsives and sexual addicts (Carnes, 1983). Even former sexual radicals, such as Rechy, have started to assert the value of celibacy. According to one report, Rechy has said, 'Philosophically, I'm unbudged. But practically we have to utterly change — to adjust to death. I'm preaching abstinence for the first time in my life' (cited in Sigal, 1987). When Rechy advocates abstinence, we are surely entering the post-sexual age!

But this is a minority view. Very early in the debates, gay activists urged the adoption of 'safer sex' and the sex positive approach to AIDS. Maas (1983) writing in the *New York Native* has argued,

> Do not waste valuable energies on negative reactions to sex. Now more than ever, ignorance, arrogance and hypocrisy about sex are to be repudiated. If anything, be more genuinely affirmative about your sexuality. At the same time you can respect without contradiction that we are dealing with a public health emergency in the form of a very serious apparently new disease that appears to be sexually transmitted. Know what the risks are and how they can be minimized. (p. 23)

The 'safe sexers' have provided the most innovative responses, but ones that are not widely known yet outside the gay community. A new language of sexual experience that advocates bodily pleasure without the exchange of bodily fluids is in the making. First suggested by Berkowitz and Callen (1983) in the publication *How to Have Sex in an Epidemic*, 'safer sex' soon became the organizing theme of gay health campaigns throughout the world. In many ways 'safer sex' is an attempt to deal with the negative meanings of AIDS — the 'stop sex' view — by maintaining positive images of sexualities and being innovative about sexual practice. For some, the emphasis is placed on *safer*, with all sexual practices being classified as high, medium or low risk activities. Despite enormous problems in measuring changes in sexual behaviour (a point clearly made by Coxon in his contribution to this book), there are signs that many gay men have indeed decreased their high-risk sexual practices (McKusick *et al.*, 1985;

Capital Gay, 1986). But for others the emphasis is placed on *sex*, with the task of eroticizing 'safer sex'; of keeping the body erotic whilst 'playing safe'. In North America, this has meant a proliferation of new sexual practices — 'telephone sex', 'jerk-off groups', 'eroticizing the condom', 'safe sex porn' and 'new styles of bodily intimacy' are all establishing themselves (Taylor, 1984; Preston, 1984; Preston and Swann, 1987).

What all this means for non-gay communities is still far from clear; penetrative, procreative sex is high risk sex if the virus is implicated, and this could mean the need for heterosexuals to copy these newer styles of gay non-procreative sexualities and foresaking the traditional view that sex must involve 'fucking'. If this is so, what consequences may this have for the birth rate in coming years?

At present, though, even in the gay community and certainly in the heterosexual one, these debates sound academic for many people who may not have sensed the message of AIDS and may remain 'fuckers'. Others may have sensed the message, but refused to countenance its relevance for them — AIDS is, after all, what happens to other people. A few may have actually grasped the message yet wilfully continue to pursue high risk activity.

These debates are complex and constantly shifting ground. New sexual meanings linked to AIDS are slowly emerging everywhere in a process by which a myriad of sexualities are being reorganized. If the shifts of the past five years pre-figure the future, sexuality in the early twenty first century could look very different from what it was in the mid twentieth. We are in the middle of a living experiment in rewriting our sexual scripts.

The Cultural Impact of AIDS

Although 'AIDS' is shaping many areas of life, it is probably the impact it is making on the overarching culture that is most significant. For not only has it become the most talked about disease in recent history, it has also come to assume all the features of a traditional morality play: images of cancer and death, or blood and semen, of sex and drugs, of morality and retribution. A whole gallery of folk devils have been introduced — the sex crazed gay, the dirty drug abuser, the filthy whore, the blood drinking voodoo-driven black — side by side with a gallery of 'innocents' — the haemophiliacs, the blood transfusion 'victim', the new born child, even the 'heterosexual'. All of this has served to illustrate the ways in which so called 'deviance' or 'stigma' comes to mark out the moral boundaries of a particular culture and establish either a degree of closure on a particular social order or provide room for some innovations and change. The work of Douglas (1970) on *Purity and Danger*, of Erikson (1966) on witchcraft purges, and of Durkheim (1964) on the 'normal and the pathological' all anticipate the case study of AIDS as the symbol of the 1980s to clarify and establish a new order. The inchoate confusions and changes so characteristic of the 1960s and early 1970s — and so inappropriately termed permissiveness — have been squashed back into the creation of a new moral order over which the symbolic threat of AIDS hangs. It is not that AIDS has simply acted as a discrete moral panic; it is rather that it has come to serve as a most potent symbol for reaffirming the older orders that have been placed under threat in the mid-twentieth century. The political stakes around AIDS have become very high indeed.

But it goes further. For with the symbolism of AIDS has emerged a range of institutional practices that aim to increase surveillance and regulation over 'deviances' and 'sexualities', many new agencies have appeared along with many new practices that aim to keep records, classify and order, take tests, watch over, maybe brand and quarantine people on the AIDS spectrum; whilst the cries for celibacy, monogamy and safer sex are becoming deafening. Small trends can become big institutions; what has emerged in the past few years may well proliferate and extend in the coming decade — establishing firm new structures for the control of 'deviance' and 'sexuality' by the end of the century. AIDS is another sign of the widening of the net and the blurring of boundaries so vividly described by Cohen (1985); it manages to 'exclude' some people more and more firmly whilst 'including' others under whole new systems of social control (*cf* Foucault, 1978, pp. 198–9).

But it goes even further than this. I have suggested throughout this chapter that AIDS is just as much a powerful symbol as it is a powerful disease. An whilst the disease may result in tragic death, the symbol may result in equally tragic life. Scratch the surface of the stereotypical stigmas I have described, and you find the developing preconditions for the segregation of whole populations of people, for branding, quarantine and perhaps even genocide. These sound wild claims and hopefully they are. But already public opinion polls suggest the popularity of compulsory segregation; already opinion leaders have made outrageous suggestions; already attempts are being made in parts of the US to enact quarantine legislation. And these are early days.

I recall, from a different context, Arendt's (1963) fine phrase 'the banality of evil'. Speaking of Eichmann and the holocaust, her writing captures how 'normal' everyday folk can both perpetrate and collude with monstrous acts of evil. In this century alone, millions upon millions have been slaughtered by ordinary people — by you and me. Many have tried to explain this dreadful phenomenon and many more have tried to ignore it. But at the very least, stereotyped stigmatized thinking can lead us to perceive whole sections of the population as somehow sub-human. And once that happens, anything can be done to them. They may be shot in the night, bombed in their cities and sent to the gas chambers. Contemporary reactions within the context of AIDS could so easily prefigure possibilities such as these. These are dramatic statements indeed, but dramatic statements about dramatic possibilities.

This chapter has been far from easy to write. Quite apart from the difficulties of attempting to identify a wide agenda of social issues worth thinking about, and quite apart from the rapidity of social change with respect to AIDS which could make much of what has been written out of date by the time this book appears, there is a more serious problem. This flows from the paradox that whilst AIDS is a serious debilitating disease which demands concern, attention, funding, research and care, it is also a profoundly symbolic event harbouring hosts of new practices, many of which may not be quite as benign as they appear: a medical profession that may control rather than cure, a government that may regulate rather than educate, a media that may disinform rather than inform and a public that may scapegoat rather than understand.

Notes

1   There are signs that symptoms of what is now called AIDS were around at least as early as 1959 (Williams, Stretton and Leonard, 1983). Certainly a number of gay men have commented that they had noticed comparable symptoms well before the disease was officially identified. Arthur Felson (in Nungesser, 1986, p. 4, became aware of it in 1977, but 'there was no information in 1977. There was no medical information at all. I saw a friend of mine die. I remember him running around from one hospital to the other, not really getting very much of an answer'). Dennis Altman has astutely noted that the cellular basis of the immune system was only discovered by Macfarlane Burnet in 1959 and that 'the discovery of the retroviruses able to infect human cells came only at the end of the 1970s, almost at the exact same time as the first cases of AIDS were being reported' (Altman, 1986, p. 11). A disease can hardly be identified if its foundations are not known. It could be suggested, therefore, that phenomena linked to what is now called AIDS have been around for some time.

2   The literature on the 'social construction of social problems' is very considerable, and the major attempt so far to relate it to AIDS is that of Vass (1986). The key background to this theory is contained in Blumer (1971), Spector and Kitsuse (1977), Gusfield (1981), Wiener (1981) and Schneider

(1985). I have adapted aspects of this argument to an analysis of homosexuality in Plummer (1981). A valuable set of critical observations are to be found in Woolgar and Pawluck (1985). In a chapter such as this there is no space to go into the intricacies of such arguments.

3 Anyone who suggests that HIV is not the cause of AIDS is usually seen as a crank. However, there are a range of alternative theories in circulation which link it to other viruses (for example, Human B-cell Lymphotropic Virus HBLV; Epstein–Barr virus, EBV; African Swine Fever Virus, ASFV); to 'virulent immunosuppressant spirochaetes', syphilis; to co-factors which range from sleeping sickness and malaria to toxic drug use and other sexually transmitted diseases; to prior damage to the immune system; and — still around — to germ warfare. Many of these ideas get a regular airing in *The New York Native*, but rarely appear in medical journals.

4 See, for example, two accounts in *Newsweek* on 'AIDS in Africa', 23 March 1987, p. 4; and 'Fear of Foreigners', 6 April 1987, p. 17.

5 Reported in the *Lancet*, 13 September 1986, p. 644. Amongst these are the *CDC Aids Weekly*, *AIDS and Retroviruses Update* (from Bureau of Hygiene and Tropical Diseases), *AIDS* (Gower Academic Journals), *AIDS Policy and Law* (*Baraff Publications*), *AIDS and Human Retroviruses* (Mary Ann Liebert, Inc). For a sample of one international conference (of many), see *Annals of Internal Medicine, 103, 5, November 1985*. At this conference over 3200 people attended from fifty countries; there were 700 abstracts and 418 presentations!

6 I am ignoring here the work of other 'death theorists' like Ernest Becker as well as the wider 'survival' literature of people like Bruno Bettelheim — all of which provides potential insights into the AIDS crisis.

7 For a discussion of the spectrum as presented here, see for example Green and Miller, 1986, p. 50; Daniels, 1985, p. 75 and 46; Farthing, 1986 *et al.*, p. 16.

8 On the history of the gay movement, see especially D'Emilio (1983) for the USA, Weeks (1977) for the UK and Adam (1987) for a wider analysis. The shifts in the gay community are most clearly analyzed in Altman (1986) and Patton (1985). *The New York Native* started publication at roughly the same time as AIDS appeared, and each issue covers gays debates around AIDS in enormous detail — so detailed it is popularly known as The New York Review of Aids! Much of it is however deeply polemical.

References

ADAM, B. (1987) *The Rise of a Gay and Lesbian Movement*, Boston, MA, Twayne.

ALTMAN, D. (1986) *AIDS and the New Puritanism*, London, Pluto Press.

ARENDT, H. (1963) *Eichmann in Jerusalem: A Report on the Banality of Evil*, New York, Viking Press.

BAYER, R. (1981) *Homosexuality and American Psychiatry: The Politics of Diagnosis*, New York, Basic Books.

BERKOWITZ, R. and CALLEN, M. (1983) *How to Have Sex in an Epidemic*: *A New Approach*, New York, News from the Front.

BETTELHEIM, B. (1986) *Surviving the Holocaust*, London, Fontana.

BLUMER, H. (1971) 'Social Problems as collective behaviour', *Social Problems*, 18. pp 298–306.

BRANDT, A. (1985) *No Magic Bullet*: *A Social History of Venereal Disease in the United States since 1880*, New York, Oxford University Press.

BRONSKI, M. (1984) *Culture Clash*: *The Making of Gay Sensibility*, Boston, MA, South End Press.

CARNES, P. (1983) *The Sexual Addiction*, Minneapolis, MN, Camp Care.

COATES, T., TEMOSHOK, L. and MANDEL, J. (1984) 'Psychological research is essential to understanding and treating AIDS', *American Psychologist*, 39, 11, pp 1309–14.

COHEN, S. (1985) *Visions of Social Control*, Cambridge, Polity Press.

CONRAD, P. and SCHNEIDER, J. (1980) *The Medicalization of Deviance*, London, C.V. Mosby.

DANIELS, V. (1985) *AIDS*. Lancaster, MTP Press.

D'EMILIO, J. (1983) *Sexual Politics, Sexual Communities*: *The Making of a Homosexual Minority in the United States, 1940–1970*, Chicago, IL, University of Chicago Press.

DEVITA, V. *et al* (1985) *AIDS*: *Etiology, Diagnosis, Treatment and Prevention*, London, Lippincott.

DINGWALL, R. (1976) *Aspects of Illness*, London, Martin Robertson.

DOUGLAS, M. (1970) *Purity and Danger*, London, Routledge and Kegan Paul.

DOYAL, L. (1979) *The Political Economy of Health*, London, Pluto Press.

DUBOS, R. (1959) *The Mirage of Health*: *Utopias, Progress and Biological Change*, London, Harper and Row.

DURKHEIM, E. (1964) *The Rules of Sociological Method*, New York, Free Press.

EDELMAN, E. (1977) *Political Language*: *Words that Succeed and Policies that Fail*, London, Academic Press.

EHRENREICH, B. *et al* (1986) *Remaking Love*: *The Feminization of Sex*, New York, Anchor.

ERIKSON, K. (1966) *Wayward Puritans*, London, Wiley.

FABREGA, H. and MANNING, P. (1972) 'Disease, illness and deviant careers' in SCOTT, R. and DOUGLAS, J. (Eds.) *Theoretical Perspectives on Deviance*, New York, Basic Books.

FARTHING, C. *et al* (1986) *A Colour Atlas of AIDS*, London, Wolfe Medical.

FELDMAN, D. and JOHNSON, T. (Eds.) (1986) *Social Dimensions of AIDS*, New York, Praeger.

FORSTEIN, M. (1984) 'The psychosocial impact of the Acquired Immune Deficiency Syndrome', *Seminars in Oncology*, 11, 1. pp 72–82.

FOUCAULT, M. (1978) *Discipline and Punish*, London, Allen Lane.

FREIDSON, E. (1970) *Profession of Medicine*: *A Study of the Sociology of Applied Knowledge*, New York, Dodd, Mead and Co.

GAGNON, J. and SIMON, W. (1973) *Sexual Conduct*, Chicago, IL, Aldine.

GOFFMAN, E. (1963) *Stigma*: *Notes on the Management of Spoiled Identity*. Harmondsworth, Penguin Books.

GREEN, J. and MILLER, D. (1986) *AIDS*: *The Story of a Disease*, London, Grafton.

GUSFIELD, J. (1981) *The Culture of Public Problems*, Chicago, IL, University of Chicago Press.

HUTTON-WILLIAMS, L. (1983) 'Deconstructing a syndrome: AIDS', *Gay Information*, 13, pp 30–8.

ILLICH, I. (1975) *Medical Nemesis*, London, Calder and Boyars.

KINGHAM, M. (1987) 'AIDS and the case of volatile inhalants' in COXON, A.P. and GILLIGAN, J. H. (Eds.) *AIDS: The Latest Moral Panic*, University College Cardiff Monograph.

KOTARBA, J. (1983) *Chronic Pain: Its Social Dimensions*, Beverley Hills, CA, Sage.

KUBLER-ROSS, E. (1970) *On Death and Dying*, London, Tavistock.

LAURITSEN, J. and WILSON, H. (1986) *Death Rush: Poppers and AIDS*, New York, Pagan Press.

LIFTON, R. (1976) *The Life of the Self*, New York, Simon and Schuster.

LIFTON, R. (1979) *The Broken Connection*, New York, Simon and Schuster.

LOCKER, D. (1981) *Symptoms and Illness: The Cognitive Organization of Disorder*, London, Tavistock.

MAAS, L. (1983) 'Guilt and AIDS', *New York Native*, 34, pp 23–5.

MCKEOWN, T. (1979) *The Role of Medicine*, Oxford, Basil Blackwell.

MCKUSICK, L. *et al* (1985) 'AIDS and sexual behaviour reported by gay men in San Francisco', *American Journal of Public Health*, 75. 5. pp 493–6.

MCNEILL, W. (1979) *Plagues and People*, Harmondsworth, Penguin Books.

MILLER, D. and GREEN, J. (1985) 'Psychological support and counselling for patients with AIDS', *Genitourinary Medicine*, 61, pp 273–8.

MOORE, A. and LEBAROU, R. (1986) 'The case for a Haitian origin of the AIDS epidemic' in FELDMAN, D. and JOHNSON, T. (Eds.) *Social Dimensions of AIDS*, New York, Praeger.

MORIN, S. *et al* (1984) 'The psychological impact of AIDS on gay men', *American Psychologist*, 39. 1. pp 1288–93.

NAVARRO, V. (1976) *Medicine Under Capitalism*, London, Croom Helm.

NICHOLS, S. (1985) 'Psychological reactions of persons with AIDS', *Annals of Internal Medicine*, 103, pp 765–7.

NUNGESSER, L. (1986) *Epidemic of Courage: Facing AIDS in America*, New York, St Martins Press.

PATTON, C. (1985) *Sex and Germs: The Politics of AIDS*, Boston, MA, South End Press.

PEABODY, B. (1986) *The Screaming Room: A Mother's Journal of her Son's Struggle with AIDS*, San Diego, CA, Oak Tree Press.

PLUMMER, K. (Ed.) (1981) *The Making of the Modern Homosexual*, London, Hutchinson.

PLUMMER, K. (1982) 'Symbolic interactionism and sexual conduct: An emergent perspective' in BRAKE, M. (Ed.) *Human Sexual Relations*, Harmondsworth, Penguin Books.

PLUMMER, K. (1985–6) 'The culture of AIDS, The politics of AIDS, Worlds apart', *Gay Times*, May, October, February.

PORTER, R. (1986) 'Plague and panic', *New Society*. 12 December, pp 11–3.

PRESTON, J. (1984) *Hot Living: Erotic Stories about Safer Sex*, New York, Alyson Publications.

PRESTON, J. and SWANN, G. (1987) *Safe Sex*, New York, Plume.

SABATIER, R. (1986) *AIDS and the Third World*, London, Panos Institute.

SCHMIDT, C. (1984) 'The group fantasy origins of AIDS', *Journal of Psychohistory*, 12. 1. pp 37–77.

SCHNEIDER, W. (1985) 'Social problems theory: The constructionist view', *Annual Review of Sociology*. pp 209–29.

SIGAL, C. (1987) 'Love in a shadow', *The Guardian*, 7 March, p 12.

SIMON, W. and GAGNON, J. (1986) 'Sexual scripts: Permanence and change', *Archives of Sexual Behaviour*, 15, 2, pp 97–120.

SNITOW, A. (Ed.) (1986) *Desire: The Politics of Sexuality*, London, Virago.

SONTAG, S. (1983) *Illness as Metaphor*, Harmondsworth, Penguin Books.

SPECTOR, M. and KITSUSE, J. (1977) *Constructing Social Problems*, Menlo Park, CA, Cummings.

SPENCE, C. (1986) *AIDS: Time to Reclaim our Power*, London, Lifestory.

STRAUSS, A. (1975) *Chronic Illness and the Quality of Life*, London, C.V. Mosby.

SUCHMAN, E. (1965) 'Stages of illness and medical care', *Journal of Health and Social Behaviour*, 6. pp 114–28

TATCHELL, P. (1986) *AIDS: A Guide to Survival*, London, Gay Men's Press.

TAYLOR, C. (1984) 'Sexology in the age of the Acquired Immune Deficiency Syndrome', *Association of Sexologists Newsletter*, June. pp 6–8.

TUCKETT, D. (Ed.) (1976) *An Introduction to Medical Sociology*, London, Tavistock.

VANCE, C. (Ed.) (1984) *Pleasure and Danger*, London, Routledge and Kegan Paul.

VAN NESS, P. (1986) *Alternative and Holistic Health Care for AIDS and Prevention*, Washington, DC, Whitman Walker Clinic.

VASS, A. (1986) *A Plague in US*, Cambridge, Venus Academica.

WEEKS, J. (1977) *Coming Out: Homosexual Politics in Britain*, London, Quartet.

WEEKS, J. (1985) *Sexuality and its Discontents*, London, Routledge and Kegan Paul.

WELLS, N. (1986) *The AIDS Virus: Forecasting its Impact*, London, Office of Health Economics.

WHITE, E. (1980) *States of Desire: Travels in Gay America*, London. Deutsch.

WIENER, G. (1981) *The Politics of Alcoholism*, New Jersey, Transaction Books.

WILLIAMS, G., STRETTON, T. and LEONARD, J. (1983) 'AIDS in 1959?', *Lancet* 12 November.

WOOLGAR, S. and PAWLUCK, D. (1985) 'How shall we move beyond constructivism?', *Social Problems*, 33. 2. pp 159–62.

WORTMAN, C. and DUNKEL-SCHETTER, C. (1979) 'Interpersonal relationships and cancer: A theorectical analysis', *Journal of Social Issues*, 35. 1. pp 120–207.

ZOLA, I. (1972) 'Medicine as an institution of social control', *Sociological Review*, 20. 4. pp 487–504.

3
AIDS, 'Moral Panic' Theory and Homophobia

Simon Watney

Pleasure is the only thing worth having a theory about — Oscar Wilde, *The Picture of Dorian Grey*

After five years of reporting on the AIDS epidemic it is clear that British TV and Press coverage is locked into an agenda which blocks out any approach to the subject which does not conform in advance to the values and language of a profoundly homophobic culture — a culture, that is, which does not regard gay men as fully or properly human. No distinction obtains for this agenda between 'quality' and 'tabloid' newspapers, or between 'popular' and 'serious' television. *The People* is still able to report that 'AIDS is not just a gay disease — victims now include a rocketing number of heterosexual men, women and children'.[1] But note the use of the word 'just' in this context. Its report goes on to describe how 'One respectable, middle-aged housewife died recently, aged 53 — a victim of her husband's promiscuity'. He had 'slept with an AIDS-infested prostitute during a business trip to Africa'. The piece concludes that 'experts agree the AIDS plague is heading for crisis proportions in Britain', a verdict reached in the larger context of a private doctor calling for the mass quarantine of all people with AIDS.

Addressing a more upwardly mobile readership, *The Mail on Sunday* recently argued that 'The greatest danger facing Britain is not unemployment. It is not poverty. It is not even nuclear war. The greatest danger today is the growing epidemic of the killer disease AIDS.[2] Jeff Ferry reports from New York that 'The US has 25,000 cases. And, according to an official US government estimate, in five years that will have increased to 270,000 cases ... that is five times as many people in America lost in the Vietnam war. No wonder the word plague is heard with increasing frequency in the States. In New York alone there are half a million people carrying the AIDS virus — including 40,000 women. That is 10 per cent of the population. Of these 7700 have active symptoms and know they are dying. The others are simply waiting on a length of fusewire'. The article ends with the question, 'Will a country that is indifferent to the threat listen? I hope so, because I have just seen the future if we don't'.

My last example comes from a recent edition of the avowedly conservative *Daily Telegraph*. At the top of the 'Tuesday Matters' page, a statistical chart shows numbers of cases since 1982 projected through to 1990. Two large arrows sweep upwards from behind a pair of drastically feminized men, the first to the figure of '20,000 projected total of all AIDS cases by 1990', the second to the figure of '800 projected total of heterosexual victims by 1990 at today's rate of increase, which may well be conservative'.[3] The text states that 'Between 10,000 and 14,000 people in Britain could be carrying the AIDS virus'. Discussion stems from the situation of Karen and Jane, who are described as 'two young women desperately trying to face the numbing emotional consequences of their early sexual encounters. Both are infected by the AIDS virus'. Unless Britain does something now 'we will inexorably follow America, where public health officers describe "rivulets of heterosexual infection" snaking out beyond the risk groups'. The article dismisses notions of risk from casual contact with people with AIDS, and also argues against calls for mass quarantine on the grounds that sheer numbers make it unrealistic smacking 'more of the concentration camp than of rational public health'. Professor Michael Adler is quoted, calling for a publicity campaign on radio and television, pointing out that 'Everyone should know that the AIDS virus cannot cross a condom'. Of the syndrome itself, the report states that 'Like an individual disease time-bomb, the virus exerts a remote-control effect. Infections and cancers, reflecting a breakdown in the immune system, may take from weeks to years to erupt'. We also learn from an American psychologist that 'The British public is in a state of "AIDS phobia" or generalized fear, based on lack of knowledge of the disease'. Addresses and telephone numbers are provided for the College of Health AIDS Healthline, the Haemophilia Society, and the Health Education Council, but not, significantly, for The Terence Higgins Trust, which is the vector of information for gay men who are clearly the constituency most directly vulnerable to infection, and most in need of information.

All three of these reports create profound problems for our understanding of AIDS, and issues of social policy surrounding it. Thus *The People* divides up people with AIDS into two categories in a discourse of 'victims', the majority of whom are 'guilty' and a minority 'innocent'. Its report also colludes with an underlying racism and misogyny which contrasts the 'respectable' housewife with AIDS with the 'infested' African prostitute. The crucial term here is 'promiscuity', which effectively cordons off married women from independent non-monogamous female sexuality, drawing on a deep reservoir of retributive judgment which is a major characteristic of Western AIDS commentary. *The Mail on Sunday* carries this approach over into its use of statistics, by wilfully confusing the numbers of people infected by the HIV virus with those who have gone on to develop AIDS. This is an absolutely fundamental point. If we do not distinguish between those who have contracted the HIV virus, which is a disease of the blood, transmitted via direct blood to blood or blood to sexual fluid contact from the various opportunistic infections which result from damage to the body's immune-system, we will have a highly misleading picture both of AIDS and of the epidemic. Such a telescoping of HIV infection with AIDS, exemplified by lazy talk of there being an 'AIDS virus', as it is described in both *The Mail on Sunday* and *The Daily Telegraph*, actively obscures understanding of the central issues involved. The 70 per cent or so of HIV infected individuals who present no symptoms at all are hardly likely to be reassured by the information that they are 'simply waiting on the end of a fusewire', whilst the 10 per cent to 30 per cent who have developed opportunistic infections are simply shamed into being regarded as responsible for their own illnesses, or else regarded as tragically 'innocent' victims, at least if they are white, middle-class and heterosexual.

AIDS and Discourses About Sexuality

It is a commonplace of medical history that every major epidemic initially appears in a specific localized population. When *The People* reports that AIDS is not 'just a gay disease', and *The Daily Telegraph* conjures up the spectacle of 'rivulets of heterosexual infection' snaking out beyond the risk groups', it should be apparent that something very strange and significant is going on. AIDS is being used to articulate modern theories of sexuality, or what Freud called object-choice, as if the virus itself is intrinsically attracted to particular sexual constituencies and not others. We need to establish once and for all, as an urgent priority, that like any other virus, HIV is not a property or respector or persons or of groups of persons. It is simply a blood disease, against which relatively simple precautions are highly effective. That public information campaigns are unable to address this fact remains in need of explanation, together with the whole tendency to either stigmatize or entirely ignore the situation of vast majority of people with AIDS. Recent British figures describe some 533 gay men with AIDS, in relation to seventeen (presumably heterosexual) women[4]. The enormity of the displacement of attention to the situation of non-gay people with AIDS speaks volumes in itself. As one American commentator has pointed out,

> For gay men, sex, that most powerful implement of attachment and arousal, is also an agent of communion, replacing an often hostile family and even shaping politics. It represents an ecstatic break with years of glances and guises, the furtive past we left behind. Straight people have no comparable experience, though it may seem so in memory. They are never called upon to deny desire, only to defer its consummation.

He concludes that 'for heterosexuals to act as if AIDS were a threat to everyone demeans the anxiety of gay men who really are at risk, and for gay men to act as if we're all going to die demeans the anguish of those who are actually ill ... '(Goldstein, 1983). A media communications industry which can only acknowledge the existence of gay men as a target for contempt and thinly veiled hatred is unlikely to be able to address itself to the issues of sexual diversity which the AIDS epidemic requires us to face as the *sine qua non* of any effective preventative strategies which alone may prevent the spread of the HIV infection, or adequate support measures for the two million gay men in the UK who live from day to day through these terrible times with varying degrees of courage and fear, anger and grief.

The Limits of Panic

Most lesbian and gay commentators on such attitudes have favoured the influential British sociological theory of 'moral panics' for the purposes of explanation and analysis. Drawing on the 'new' criminology developed in the late 1960s, Stanley Cohen (1972) described how societies

> appear to be subject, every now and then, to periods of moral panic. A condition, episode or person emerges to become defined as a threat to societal values and interests; its nature is presented in a stylized and stereotypical fashion by the mass media; the moral barricades are manned by editors, bishops, politicians and other right-thinking people; ... Sometimes the panic passes over and is

forgotten, except in folk-lore and collective memory; at other times it has more serious and long-lasting repercussions and might produce such changes as those in legal and social policy or even in the way the society perceives itself.

Subsequent writers, of whom Stuart Hall (1978) is perhaps the most notable, have developed this general picture to embrace the entire process by which popular consent is won for measures which require a 'more than usual' exercise of regulation, particularly in domains which are tradition-ally understood in liberal philosophy to be private, and especially the home. Hall's work in particular has encouraged a 'stages' view of moral panics, leading to increasingly punitive state control, although it is important to stress that moral panics do not necessarily stem from the state itself, or any of its immediate avatars. On the contrary, what is at stake is the entire relationship between governments and other uneven and conflicting institutions addressing a supposedly unified 'general public' through the mass media. This is particularly important to bear in mind for anyone approaching the question of the representation of homosexuality in this culture, since the entire subject is already and always historically preconstituted as 'scandal'. Indeed, one of the major reasons why lesbian and gay critics were attracted to 'moral panic' theory in the first place was because it offered a corrective alternative to the then dominant school of orthodox sociological 'deviance' theory, which holds, as Jeffrey Weeks (1981) has pointed out, that sexual unorthodoxy 'is somehow a quality inherent in ... individuals, to which the social then has to respond'. For 'deviance' theorists homosexuality is itself a problem, whereas 'moral panic' theory allows us to examine some of the conditions and means whereby homosexuality is problematized.

In his most recent book Jeffrey Weeks (1986) describes how 'one of the most striking features of the AIDS crisis is that, unlike most illnesses, from the first its chief victims were chiefly blamed for causing the disease, whether because of their social attitudes or sexual practices'. He goes on to explain how 'In the normal course of a moral panic there is a characteristic stereotyping of the main actors as peculiar types of monsters, leading to an escalating level of fear and peceived threat, the taking up of panic stations and absolutist positions, and a search for symbolic, and usually imaginary solutions to the dramatized problem'. Gayle Rubin (1984) has also described moral panics as,

> the 'political moment' of sex, in which diffuse attitudes are channeled into political action and from there into social change. The white slavery hysteria of the 1950s, and the child pornography

panic of the late 1970s were typical moral panics. Because sexuality in Western societies is so mystified, the wars over it are often fought at oblique angles, aimed at phony targets, conducted with misplaced passions, and are highly, intensely symbolic. Sexual activities often function as signifiers for personal and social apprehensions to which they have no intrinsic connection. During a moral panic, such fears attach to some unfortunate sexual activity or population. The media become ablaze with indignation, the public behaves like a rabid mob, the police are activated, and the state enacts new laws and regulations. When the furore has passed, some innocent erotic group has been decimated, and the state has extended its power into new areas of erotic behaviour ... Moral panics rarely alleviate any real problem, because they are aimed at chimeras and signifiers. They draw on the pre-existing discursive structure which invents victims in order to justify treating 'vices' as crimes.

This is how Gayle Rubin, and many other commentators, have qualified what has been going on around AIDS for the last several years. However, the very longevity and continuity of AIDS commentary already presents a problem for a 'moral panic' theory, in so far as this is evidently a panic which refuses to go away, a permanent panic as it were, rather than a 'political moment'. Whilst we may find a certain initial descriptive likeness to familiar events in their description as moral panics, this does not help us to understand the constant nature of ideological supervision and non-state regulation of sexuality throughout the modern period, especially in matters concerning representation. To begin with, the idea of a moral panic may be employed to characterize *all* conflicts in the public domain where stigmatization takes place. It cannot however discriminate between different orders or different degrees of moral panic. Nor can it explain why certain types of event should be especially privileged in this way. Above all, it obscures the endless 'overhead' narrative of such phenomena, as one panic gives way to another, and different panics overlap and reinforce one another. We need to understand how some moral panics may condense a host of anxieties, focusing them on a single target object, whilst others work in tandem to produce a unified effect which is only partially present and articulated in any one of its component elements. Thus for example AIDS commentary tends to draw on a wide range of concerns about childhood sexuality, homosexuality, prostitution, pornography, drug use, and so, which heavily overdetermine all discussion of the virus. At the same time the continual reporting of sexual assaults, murders, debates on sex education in schools and so on all orchestrate the larger question of sexuality itself, as something to be understood as intrinsically dangerous.

Moral panic theory directs our attention to sites of visible intervention concerning, for example, pornography, immigration policy, or abortion, which have strong public profiles. In this respect we might think of a moral panic around AIDS in terms of stories concerning the forcible detention of people with AIDS, or the presence of gay men (by now practically synonymous with the rhetorical figure of the 'AIDS-carrier') on the Royal Yacht Britannia, and so on and so forth. But this encouragement to think of AIDS commentary primarily if not exclusively in terms of *excess* does not help us make sense, for example, of government inaction, or the hysterical modesty of politicians from Mrs. Thatcher downwards who have been against the provision of explicit safer-sex advice on television or in newspaper 'public information' campaigns. Their actions are far more damaging and dangerous in the long run than all the ravings of Fleet Street, since they effectively condemn thousands of people to ignorance about the very strategies by which lives may be saved. Just as the Centers for Disease Control in the United States have consistently refused to fund sexually explicit educational materials, so until recently the British government is effectively sentencing countless gay to men to death. As Ann Guidici Fettner (1986) concludes, 'AIDS education should have been started the moment it was realized that the disease is sexually transmitted'. In this situation it is difficult but vitally important to recognize that from the perspective of the state gay men are regarded in their entirety as a disposable population.

Classical moral panic theory interprets representations of specific 'scandals' as events which appear and then disappear, having run their ideological course. Such a view makes it difficult to theorize representation as a site of *permanent* ideological struggle and contestation between rival pictures of the world. We do not in fact watch the unfolding of discontinuous and discrete 'moral panics', but rather the mobility of ideological confrontations across the entire field of industrialized communications. This is most markedly the case in relation to those images which handle and evaluate the meanings of the human body, where rival and incompatible institutions and values are involved in a ceaseless and remorseless struggle to discover and disclose its supposedly universal 'human' truth. Hence the intensity of struggle to define the meanings of AIDS, with the virus being used by all and sundry as a kind of glove-puppet from the mouth of which different interest groups speak their values. AIDS, however, has no single 'truth' of its own, but becomes a powerful condensor for a great range of social, sexual and psychic anxieties. This is why it is better to think in terms of AIDS commentary, rather than assuming the existence of a coherent univocal 'moral panic' on the subject. We are here considering the circulation of symbols, of the raw materials from which human subjectivity is constructed. AIDS has been mobilized to embody a variety of perceived threats to individual and social stability, organized around th spectacle of illicit sex and physical corruption. It has been used to stabilize the figure of the heterosexual family unit which remains the central image in our society with which individuals are endlessly invited to identify their collective interests and their very core of being.

The Instrumental Family

As Foucault (1979) and others have argued, we need however to recognize that the image of the threatened and vulnerable family is a central motif in a society like ours for which the family is not simply a given object, but is rather an instrument of social policy. What AIDS commentary reveals is the ongoing crisis surrounding the representation of the family in a culture in which only a minority of citizens actually occupy its conventional space at any given moment in time. Familial ideology is thus obliged to fight a continual rearguard action in order to disavow the social and sexual diversity of a culture which can never be adequately pictured in the traditional guise of the family. Those who threaten to expose the ideological operations of familialism will inevitably be castigated as 'enemies' of the family, which is pictured as under constant threat.

Thus Sir Rhodes Boyson, the Minister for Local Government, recently grouped together feminists, single-parent families, and 'the fashion of the flaunting and propagation of homosexuality and lesbianism as anti-family and anti-life'.[5] In such a view, lesbians and gay men cannot be regarded as constituencies within a pluralist society. Rather, they are to be identified as prime agents of anti-social, and even extra-human danger.

It is clear that the categories which hold together the public profile of familialism — notions of 'decency', 'respectability', 'manliness', 'innocence', and so on — are primarily defensive, in so far as they work to protect individuals from the partially acknowledged fact of diversity. Hence the repetitive nature of moral panics, their fundamentally *serial* nature, and the wide range of tones and postures which they can assume 'on behalf' of the national family unit. The organization of desire in all its forms into the narrow channels of modern sexual identities ensures that the presence of 'enemies' is felt everywhere, within the self, and from without.

This is why there is such a dramatic disparity between the lived experience of people with AIDS, and the model of contagion which they are made to embody. We are not living through a distinct, coherent 'moral panic' concerning AIDS, a panic with a linear narrative and the prospect of closure. On the contrary, we are witnessing the ideological manoevres which unconsciously 'make sense' of this accidental triangulation of disease, sexuality, and homophobia. Hence the obsession of AIDS commentary with the distinction between supposedly 'innocent' and 'guilty' victims, and the total inability to distinguish between infectious and contagious illness. AIDS commentary rarely troubles to separate the question of HIV infection from individual opportunistic infection, preferring to talk of 'AIDS-carriers' and an 'AIDS-virus'. What we should recognize is that such telescoping of medical issues indicates a collapsing together of ideological concerns, which transform AIDS into a *malade imaginaire* — the viral personification of unorthodox deregulative desire, dressed up in the ghoulish likeness of degeneracy.

Hence, in the popular imagination of AIDS, we come close to the core of modern familial identities and social policy for which the perverse maps out the boundaries of the legitimate social order. This is why we need to be able to analyze the relations of contingency, analogy and substitution between phenomena which moral panic theory obliges us to think of as discrete and unconnected. Sociology obliges us to think of individual 'moral panics' around drugs, video films, football hooliganism, and so on, because it regards the family as 'a point of departure' rather than a product of complex negotiation between different institutional and discursive formations. Moral panics do not 'reflect' something we should think of as 'the social': on the contrary, they constitute the ground on which 'the social' emerges, in the words of Jacques Donzelot (1979), as 'a concrete space of intelligibility of the family' in which 'it is the social that suddenly looms as a strange abstraction'.

It is thus particularly unhelpful to think of AIDS commentary as a moral panic which somehow makes gay men into monsters, since that is an intrinsic effect of the medicalization of morality which accompanied the emergence of the modern categories of sexuality in the course of the last 200 years. What AIDS commentary does is to elide the virus and its presenting symptoms with the dominant cultural meanings of those constituencies in which it has emerged — black Africans, injecting drug users, prostitutes, and of course gay men. In this manner 'the social' is ever more narrowly confined within familial definitions and values, with the family being scrutinized ever more closely for physical symptoms of moral dissent. The sheer range and variety of AIDS commentary should alert us to the danger of any attempt to explain it in terms of any single, primary and all-determining causes. This however is precisely the tendency of the many lesbian and gay commentators who rely upon the notion of 'homophobia' as if this were an adequate, sufficient, and self-evident explanatory category. The term itself was first defined if not coined by George Weinberg (1973) in the immediate wake of Gay Liberationist politics in the early 1970s as 'a disease' and 'an attitude held by many non-homosexuals and perhaps by the majority of homosexuals in countries where there is discrimination against homosexuality'. For its inception, it uncomfortably straddled both the situation of all social and psychic aspects of attitudes towards homosexuality, as well as both homosexual and heterosexual identities. In effect the notion simply reversed the sociological and psychiatric tendencies to pathologize all forms of homosexual identity and desire as symptoms of either 'deviance' or 'perversion'.

This confusion of social and psychic factors has dogged the history of the term's usage ever since. Thus Cindy Patton's (1986) recent notion of 'erotophobia' faithfully duplicates all the problems of the original term, being defined as

> the terrifying irrational reaction to the erotic which makes individuals and societies vulnerable to psychological and social control in cultures where pleasure is strictly categorized and regulated. Each component of sexuality — sexual practice, desire, and sexual identity — constitutes a particular type of relationship between the individual and society, providing gripping opportunities for different forms of erotophobic repression.

Conclusion

Elsewhere, I have attempted to separate out some of the central strands within the hysterical dimensions of homosexual stigmatization.[6] In this context though, I would like to return to the question of *systematic misinformation* concerning medical aspects of AIDS with which I began this chapter. Both doctors and journalists share a common professional training which massively privileges the family as the central term of social intelligibility. That doctors should be in the foreground of calls for the mass quarantine of people with AIDS is not in the least surprising, given the 'protective' identity which they are taught in medical school and in medical practice. Medicine remains perhaps the most difficult profession in which to 'come out' in the UK, and many young doctors have been ostracized and held back in their careers for no other reason. Indeed, the National Health Service itself addresses a 'national' population which signally and conspicuously fails to recognize the existence of lesbians and gay men as a fundamental constituency within the nation, let alone our specific medical needs. Effectively, 'national' medicine thereby becomes 'heterosexual' medicine, as is evident from the dramatic under-funding of hospitals and clinics as the AIDS epidemic proceeds to escalate. This is equally apparent from the inability of a medically constituted public information campaign to directly address the actual diversity of sexual practice with the 'public' which they supposedly addressing. Whilst the avoidance of a forbidden object is certainly a sign of phobia, we should remember that phobic avoidance is focussed not on what it is unconsciously afraid, but on displaced symbols of the terrifying object.

Some degrees of phobic response to homosexuality would seem to be the inevitable result of the psychic violence involved in the process which attempts to homogenize all children into the 'correct' identities of adult heterosexuality. But the notion of homophobia precisely avoids the whole question of how desire operates to motivate particular sexual behaviours. At the same time it serves to further regulate and reinforce the workings of modern sexual categories by seemingly forcing together all the varieties of homosexual desire and identity into a monolithic totality, faced by an equally monolithic heterosexuality. Whatever else might be said to characterize homophobia or erotophobia, the fact remains that their signs are understood to be expulsive and aggressive, rather than avertive and defensive.

Thus any approach to AIDS commentary rooted in a critique of homophobia is unlikely to be able to come to grips with subtle questions of metaphor, displacement, repetition, substitutions or absences, privileging instead the most violent physical and verbal abuse of people with AIDS, which in any case is relatively transparent in terms of ordinary liberal 'civil rights' analysis. The questions of why the HIV virus continues to be treated as if it were contagious and transmissable by casual contact, proves stubbornly resistant to the explanatory schemes provided either by 'moral panic' theory, or notions of a unified homophobia. Both in effect offer little more than 'false-consciousness' accounts of how different desiring constituencies perceive and evaluate one another, together with a latent functionalism which glimpses either a unified purposive state or a coherent collectivity of 'heterosexuality' at work behind social and psychic attitudes to AIDS.

Nonetheless, it is probably more helpful than not at this moment in time to retain the notion of homophobia at least as a collective term, referring to the entire range of interacting institutions, discourses and psychic processes which align AIDS with homosexuality as if by essence. This argument is supported by the probability that much hostility towards homosexuality is indeed phobic in origin, in so far as it stems from the threatening return to consciousness of desires and fantasies concerning the human body which can never be completely contained and successfully repressed within the narrow compass of heterosexual identities which defensively equate sexuality with sexual reproduction. The real 'threat' comes not from lesbians or gay men, but from the destabilization of conscious heterosexual identities from within themselves.

In this respect we can recognize that the most frequently encountered characteristic of AIDS commentary is projection, defined by Leo Bersani (1977) as 'a frantic defence against the return of dangerous images and sensations to the surface of consciousness; therefore, the individual urgently needs to maintain that certain representations or affects belong to the world and not to the self'. In this manner we can begin to account for the ways in which AIDS is invariably made to carry a fantastic supplement which both precedes and exceeds any actual medical issues. In the same way we can chart the compulsive displacements which add up to the public meanings of AIDS, the scattering of themes and motifs across the entire field of public representation. To fail to notice the systematic connections between contemporary campaigns around sex education, procreation, children's sexuality and AIDS, by classifying them as separate and autonomous 'moral panics' is as dangerous today as any temptation to regard them all as no more than epiphenomena related to a unified and totally recalcitrant homophobia.

Notes

1 OWEN, J. and ROSEN, C. (1986) 'Put AIDS victims in holiday camps: Doctor's shock remedy'. *The People*, 28 September.
2 FERRY, J. (1986) 'AIDS: The chilling last-chance warning for Britain'. *The Mail on Sunday*, 12 October.
3 DOYLE, C. (1986) 'AIDS: It does affect us all', *The Daily Telegraph*, 15 September.
4 *The Daily Telegraph*, 2 December 1986.
5 HENKE, D. (1986) 'Boyson condemns "evil" single parents'. *The Guardian*. 10 October.
6 WATNEY, S. (1987) *Policing Desire: Pornography, AIDS and the media*, London, Comedia, Methuen.

Simon Watney

References

BERSANI, L. (1977) *Baudelaire and Freud*, Los Angeles, CA, University of California Press.

COHEN, S. (1972) *Folk Devils and Moral Panics: The Creation of the Mods and Rockers*, London, Martin Robertson.

DONZELOT, J. (1979) *The Policing of Families: Welfare versus the State*, London, Hutchinson.

FOUCAULT, M. (1979) 'On governmentality', *Ideology and Consciousness*, 6, pp. 5–21.

GIUDICI FETTNER, A. (1986) 'Is the CDC dying of AIDS?', *Village Voice*, 21, 40, 7 October.

GOLDSTEIN, R. (1983) 'Heartsick: Fear and loving in the gay community', *Village Voice*, 28, 26, 28 June.

HALL, S. *et al* (1978) *Policing The Crisis*, London, Macmillan.

PATTON, C. (1986) *Sex and Germs: The Politics of AIDS*, Boston, MA, South End Press.

RUBIN, G. (1984) 'Thinking sex: Notes for a radical theory of the politics of sexuality' in VANCE, C (Ed.) *Pleasure and Danger: Exploring Female Sexuality*, London, Routledge and Kegan Paul.

WEEKS, J. (1981) *Sex, Politics and Society: The Regulation of Sexuality Since 1800*, London, Longman.

WEEKS, J. (1986) *Sexuality*, London, Tavistock.

WEINBERG, G. (1973) *Society and the Healthy Homosexual*, New York, Doubleday.

4
Illness, Metaphor and AIDS

Keith Alcorn

This chapter seeks to situate Human Immunodeficiency Virus (HIV) infection and Acquired Immune Deficiency Syndrome (AIDS) within normative discourses on health and illness in order to understand the ways in which AIDS has been represented as a modern disease as well as the uses to which it has been put in identifying new standards of health — a crucial function of the medical disciplinary apparatus. Attention will also be given to analyzing some of the ways in which AIDS is challenging the power relations that presently avail within mainstream medical practice.

In order to do this, I will first examine in general terms the ways in which health and illness have been used as metaphors by which to express anxieties about the place of the body in the social order. I will then look at some of the ways in which AIDS has been made to perform a similar function, both in relation to society as a whole and with respect to modern medical practice in particular. Finally, I will try to identify some of the challenges which self-help and community-based interventions with respect to HIV infection and AIDS pose for dominant medical orthodoxies.

Metaphor and the Social Construction of Illness

Sontag's (1983) book *Illness and Metaphor*, which was written following her own treatment for cancer, and in which she analyzes the imagery surrounding cancer and tuberculosis, has been highly influential in enabling us to begin to appreciate the processes by which illness is constructed in the popular imagination. In it, she identifies, amongst other things, the metaphorical uses to which illness and disease may be put in 'making sense' of prevailing social arrangements. In many respects, her work echoes that of Foucault (1973) who, in *The Birth of the Clinic*, argues for there being a typical disease of the age: one which reflects central pre-occupations with the social order and the place of the body within it. Foucault suggests,

> diseases vary from one period ... to another. In the Middle Ages, a time of war and famine, the sick were subject to fear and exhaustion (apoplexy and hectic fever); but in the sixteenth and seventeenth century, a period of relaxation, of feeling for one's country and of the obligations that such a feeling involves, egotism returned and lust and gluttony became more widespread (venereal diseases, congestion of the viscera and of the blood); in the eighteenth century, the search for pleasure was carried over into the imagination; one went to the theatre, read novels and grew excited, one stayed up at night and slept during the day (hysteria, hypochondria, nervous diseases). (p. 33)

This way of understanding the relationship between disease and civilization holds true even today and the inconsistencies associated with it remain part of the taken for granted reality of those who seek to regulate behaviour through the institutionalized practices of modern medicine.

But diseases can also have pseudo-revolutionary metaphors attached to them. Tuberculosis, for example, had strong associations with the Romantic movement during the early nineteenth century. Although its associations with gentility (as a smarter social disease than gout) had already been established by the 1770s in England, in the nineteenth century tuberculosis became known as a disease of languor, pallor, invalidity and withdrawal from the world that belied a spirit against the prevailing atmosphere of the time. In the great century of accumulation and imperialism, the Romantic response was to invest a wasting disease with the power not only to represent the thwarting and conversion of individualistic, romantic love into something corrosive, but also to speak of superior nature not long for this base world. Tuberculosis could be cured, it was thought, only by confinement or travel, preferably to far away places, and always away from the city, as well as by removal from the daily routine and bodily submission to a set of rules laid down by the newly powerful medical profession.

It was thought by many in the early nineteenth century that tuberculosis made one 'interesting'. Interesting, because the disease individualized and set the patient apart. Because tuberculosis did not seem to strike at a community or race or family as an epidemic, but at individuals, it became a vehicle for the production of the self. The languor and thinness associated with fashion and grace in our century are in fact the legacy of nineteenth century consumptives. Continuous coughing, 'far from making me look ugly ... gives me an air of langour that is very becoming', said one Parisian woman at the time (Sontag, 1983, p. 33).

Tuberculosis was also thought to derive from undirected passion. William Blake wrote in *The Proverbs of Hell* that 'He who desires but acts not, breeds pestilence'. Tuberculosis was seen by the Romantic movement as 'a failure of the desiring subject to realize the ideals of vitality and perfect spontaneity that their individualistic philosophy demanded' (Sontag, 1983, p. 49). It was in fact a disease of the will. At the time, death from tuberculosis was believed to be relatively painless: one expired, rather than died in agony with a stench on the breath as was so frequently the case with other diseases.

In contrast, cancer has been widely portrayed as a disease that requires not rest and isolation (for it is not contagious) but a fight to what will probably be an agonizing death. Cancer did not make one interesting but 'ashamed' — being indicative of the moral predisposition of one's character. Variously considered to derive from failure and lack of expression, from isolation and hopelessness; in the nineteenth century cancer was widely believed to have its origins in overcrowding, bereavement and the burdens of work and home — anxieties associated with a more individualistic, atomized society.

Sontag points out that ideas about cancer and tuberculosis express a complex set of ideas about energy and feeling, strength and weakness that derive from concern about the place of these attributes within the social order. Fantasies about tuberculosis in the last century thereby reflect early capitalist concerns with 'consumption' in more than one sense. The body (like a mismanaged economy) wastes away when its energy is spent recklessly or when desire is unchecked. In imagery relating to cancer, on the other hand, we find unregulated growth and an repressed desire (the body is 'hijacked' by 'subversive' cells with a life of their own, often, it is thought, as a result of the repression of feeling and energy) that is symptomatic of the concerns and the stresses within a society that seeks to manufacture and contain desire through the market.

Diseases can also be used as metaphors for what is feared. In the popular imagination, 'corruption, decay, pollution, anomie and weakness' become particularly attached to diseases 'whose causality is murky and for which treatment is ineffectual' (*ibid*, p. 62). This process has allowed leprosy, syphilis as well as cancer to identify decay, pollution and disorder. Ideologies of blood, race and nation have particularly favoured syphilis as a symbol of moral and physical decline (Bland and Mort, 1983), but this illness with clear origins soon gave way to cancer, 'in the service of a simplistic view of the world turned paranoid' (Sontag, 1983, p. 73).

But it is to the issue of illness and the individual that we must return. In her own writing, Sontag (*ibid*, p. 76) suggests that tuberculosis and cancer were instrumental in proposing 'new, critical standards of individual health' and in expressing 'a sense of dissatisfaction with society as such'. This usage became prevalent only during the eighteenth century as an important shift in the understanding and treatment of illness took place. In consequence, it began to be widely accepted that diseases were the *product* of social disorder. If only society could be made more orderly, the health of the populace would improve. The unspoken point of all this was the recognition that the wealth of nations depended on the well-being and controlled reproduction of the workforce. The social organization of health thereby became intimately linked to that of the economy (Doyal with Pennell, 1979).

Concurrent with these changes, however, were others in response to the expanding activities of the medical profession. Until the nineteenth century, doctors did not seek to *cure an illness* but rather, to *restore the patient to health*. It was only after a century of meticulous observation, achieved largely through the dissection of the human body, that the identification of specialized pathologies could take place and certain standards of normal functioning for the body could be postulated. Following this, the medical profession became a largely *disciplinary* force alongside other concurrently emerging professions and institutions — criminology, the prison, the asylum, the factory school, the orphanage, and later sexology. This intricately structured disciplinary apparatus could not operate by coercion, but depended on the widespread acceptance of individual standards as well as an emphasis on character, personality and normality (McGrath, 1984).

During the nineteenth century, sexuality in particular became a subject of scientific enquiry, establishing new concepts of normality based not on relations between the sexes but within the family, which thereafter became the central arena of sexual discipline. The influence of this disciplinary movement for modern understandings of illness and the responses made to it cannot be underestimated. Besides establishing much of the twentieth century medical agenda, it also framed contemporary discourse about illness by individualizing and pathologizing its correlates. In the case of cancer, this has taken place largely through psychology (identifying the factors that predispose a person to cancer has been a favourite preoccupation of psychologists and therapists for years). In the case of AIDS, as we shall see, this task has been largely accomplished through links to homosexuality and sexual promiscuity.

Making Use of AIDS

AIDS differs from diseases such as tuberculosis and cancer both medically and in terms of its social construction, and its metaphorical uses have been complex. Nevertheless, it has its origins in the same hinterland of doubt and terror as these two diseases. Larry Kramer's play *The Normal Heart* is important for the way in which it charts the syndrome's first steps out of that land, a phenomenon experienced by all who have seen the play as one which fills those who witness it with hideous doubt.

In the early years of the epidemic, knowledge about AIDS was limited and uncertain: it was known to affect *homosexuals*, it was known to *kill* and it was known to be *spreading rapidly*. As we shall see, these 'facts' were paramount in setting the parameters for subsequent representations of the syndrome. Subsequently, it became clearer that the disease was spread by sexual contact and a virus was identified and isolated from blood and semen. It is now widely accepted that anal intercourse, formerly the erotic mainspring of gay culture if one is to accept reductionist rhetoric, is one of the most effective means of transmitting the virus. In the period between the identification of AIDS and the proposal of a provisional 'solution' to the problem through safer sex, a chain of very specific associations came to be linked to the syndrome. These will not drop lightly, and they betray a disturbing complex of ideas about homo-sexuality, homophobia and sexual behaviour that have been largely undebated by gay men.

First, if AIDS is a disease of sex, then sex must be equated with death. This, of course, is an old idea: one partly rooted in the economistic metaphors of the nineteenth century, when English slang equated coming with *spending* and the French called orgasm *le petit mort*, but the mystical associations of sex with death are more ancient than this. In astrology, the eight house of the zodiac and the sign of Scorpio correspond both to the transformative power of sexuality and to transformation through death. In October 1984 it was pointed out by the *New York Native's* astrologer that AIDS was a highly appropriate disease to appear when Pluto, the ruler of Scorpio, was in its own sign; linked as it is with death, sexually transmitted diseases and the so-called darker side of life and the psyche. There is much dormant imagery here for a mystical and fearful response to the current health crisis.

But this is not all. Sodomy too was once punishable by death in many European countries, and remains illegal in some American states: a sentence of death for the transgression of supposedly immutable moral laws. The AIDS epidemic seems also to have provided a biological justification for the guilt and lack of self-esteem that gay men have all to often been encouraged to feel by the rest of society. Some scientists have been heard to wonder whether gay men might not after all, have a genetic predisposition to life-threatening disease. Perhaps their supposedly weaker characters were reflected in a weaker immune system! Immune Overload theory, which suggested that too much drinking, fucking, semen, STDs, drugs, antibiotics, poppers or weekends on Fire Island were to blame for a compromised immune system (choose your lifestyle, choose your death), was so widely accepted in the early years of the epidemic that it must have nurtured many a seed of self-doubt and reproach in the minds of gay men.

AIDS: The Prisoner of Sex

But most significant of all was the swift realization that AIDS was a disease of sex. Since the nineteenth century the belief has grown that sex is perfectable; that there can exist a pure form of sex unfettered by the repressions of society and psyche. A whole new arena of discourse, devoted solely to sex rather than to its effects on the body, the soul or the productive capacity of the individual, made it a subject of paramount importance in society. Ironically, the same processes gave rise to a set of new disciplinary apparatuses that developed specially to tend to the sexual subject. Progressively within the twentieth century, sexologists and venereologists have together exercised a new and positive power over people that has been highly influential in framing modern discourse about sexual activity and desire.

Sex has served political and moral purposes for gay men too. After the Second World War, self-identified homosexual communities grew steadily in Western countries with a corresponding increase in gay sexual activity. In the 1970s, bath-houses and backrooms, environments which Foucault called 'laboratories of sex' emerged widely in US to provide a self-regulated arena for public sex — a form of activity that at the time promoted unease among gays and heterosexuals alike. This same period saw an increased incidence of Hepatitis B, Herpes and Amoebiasis as well as the more common sexually transmitted diseases within sections of the gay community, phenomena which many attributed to the new modalities of sexual practice that these environments facilitated. Inevitably AIDS too came to be depicted as a consequence of this 'sexual revolution', and we must consider the beliefs inherent in this claim if we are to understand the subsequent panic with which the syndrome has been greeted outside the gay community.

Foucault (1979) and Weeks (1985) have made important attempts to explain why sex is so important, so separate from the other human 'attributes'. They conclude that it is because our culture believes that sex speaks the truth about ourselves, that it expresses the essence of our being, that it has become the subject of such furious debate. Any concern about the social order is inevitably projected onto this essence, and through this sexuality becomes both an anxious metaphor and a subject of social control.

Polemicizing about sex is therefore never the prerogative of the progressive, even in a society that believes itself to be comparatively liberal. It is equally an instrument of normalization, of repression and recuperation. Thus, concerns about 'sexual revolution', the rising tide of 'permissiveness' and the 'threat to the family' expressed throughout the 1960s and 1970s, are a sign of more hidden anxieties about strength and weakness in the social order, about the future of existing social arrangements. This sense of crisis, whether one describes it as an extended moral panic or a new millenarianism, the rise of the New Right or the collapse of an illusory consensus, has provided a fertile source of ideas and images for the ways in which AIDS has been described and defined.

In this respect, the arguments espoused by the moral majority are well known. From the most hysterical polemic of Lyndon LaRouche who, amongst other things, has campaigned for the denial of specific employment rights for people with HIV infection and/or AIDS, to the insidious asides of politicians here in Britain, all is far from well. Such views are excellently documented in recent books by Weeks (1985) and Patton (1985). Rather than focus on these, however, I will seek here to address another modern (and more liberal) set of arguments about AIDS: those which seek to locate the syndrome as a *beast out of control* in a *world turned nasty*.

Amis (1985) has recently suggested in an article entitled 'Making sense out of AIDS' that AIDS is a disease of sex which places its victims at the 'forefront, the very pinnacle of human suffering'. This view, which suggests that the problem is so desperate that there is very little that can be done about it, recruits AIDS as a device by which to curtail the 'sexual revolution' (something which Amis himself describes as 'the liberation of coitus, the rutting revolution'). In arguing this case, Amis remarks that 'Being gay — which Americans call a lifechoice and which we might perhaps call a destiny — is a different proposition now'. Presuming to speak for gay identity is one thing, but to refer to it in terms of *destiny* is quite another. The word suggests predetermination, the elect, the damned, the judged. It has an uncomfortable association with the rhetoric of puritanism and judgment, of resignation and powerlessness.

Fundamentalist Christian magazines such as *The Plain Truth* have already made the connection between AIDS and judgment. According to their analysis, the last days will be preceded by plague, and AIDS is clearly a judgment on those most deserving of groups: homosexuals, drug users and prostitutes. As Sontag (1983): has commented, 'nothing is more punitive than to give a disease a meaning — invariably a moralistic one' (p. 62).

But all diseases have meaning, either to their sufferers or to those around them. But these meanings are generated within specific sociohistorical contexts. As such, they often reflect the nature of power relations within these settings, be these between the citizen and the state, between nations, between classes or between the sexes. If AIDS is a metaphor for the current crisis within sexual relations, then it simply represents another deeper set of social anxieties.

Considerable energy and ingenuity is needed to bind together the discourses on sexuality, practices, rights, power, privacy, gender, social relations and deviancy into which AIDS has intervened. A particularly prevalent way of doing this has been to assume that gay liberation was essentially little more that a *politics of lifestyle*. Media representations of AIDS have repeatedly identified lifestyle as a cause of illness (usually in the guise of Immune Overload theory) since lifestyle speaks contemptuously of character in these readings. An ostentatious overconsumption of sexual partners and drugs can be seen in recent media portrayals of gay life in the fast lane that emphasize the message 'I deserved it'. These representations seek to establish a character particularly susceptible to AIDS — feckless, self-indulgent, guilt-ridden — and they are not confined to the straight press.

Indeed, perhaps the most controversial writing on the subject is that by Larry Kramer, who in 1981 wrote a passionate article calling on gay men to stop having sex or be doomed. Kramer was subsequently accused of anti-eroticism, gay homophobia and scaremongering. His play *The Normal Heart* is in part a protest at the belligerence with which many gays have rejected his perhaps retributive view of AIDS, which he saw as the inevitable consequence of the gay lifestyle.

'To dress for sex now seems an act of hubris, if not a mark of susceptibility to AIDS … the very process of AIDS awareness has created its own incipient pathology' wrote Richard Goldstein in 1983, remarking on the sudden shift in codes that had established a lifestyle and character susceptible to death (p. 9). Following AIDS, there have been dramatic changes in sexual behaviour within the gay community. But have there been corresponding changes in sexual imagery, and are there new 'safe' characters and identities on the way? A cursory scan of the gay erotica currently available abroad will reveal that it is the moustache that has gone and the healthy vigorous youth who has once again emerged as the object of our desire. There is also a more intense eroticization of sex and health together in the imagery we find in magazines, books and videos, with more scenarios moving to the gym, the pool and the track, and away from the locker-room, the shower and the baths. Do such transformations represent a valorization of the active body, or are they simply a reflection of changing leisure patterns, both in response to AIDS and diverse opportunities? Do they establish characters that are safe and healthy, whilst simultaneously reproducing an unsafe, undesirable sexuality? Within this chapter it is not possible to explore in any detail the complex changes in gay iconography that have occurred in the last few years, but I would suggest that there are certain images irrevocably linked to AIDS by virtue of their association with clone culture. Many of these are being widely rejected as part of a developing AIDS consciousness and as part of a more pervasive transform ation within gay erotics.

For many gay men, the body is chiefly a source of pleasure; its position in the social order as a subject of discipline has largely been ignored except within the context of debates about pleasure. The problem of how gay men could relate both to the medical profession and to that profession's view of the body remained largely unchallenged throughout the 1970s in America. Discussion of these issues largely took place in those circles which had already rejected the commercial gay scene anyway. It was not until the arrival of AIDS that the need to reclaim personal power and bodily efficacy within the context of medical treatment (and particularly in terminal illness) began to become a crucial issue. Unlike women, who have been the subjects of widespread infantilization and regulation by institutionalized medical practice (most notably with regard to reproduction and childbirth), many gay men have remained largely ignorant of the power relations that pervade modern medical treatment except when attending an STD clinic.

AIDS: An Illness of Difference

Some researchers believe that the more unsafe sex one has with infected partners, the greater the risk of infection. Others believe that one chance encounter is enough to become HIV antibody-positive. These are widely held viewpoints and have contributed to an certain understanding of AIDS as a *disease of lifestyle* by simultaneously suggesting that one can top-up the levels of HIV in the body (and that one therefore becomes ill because of wanton promiscuity) and that one shot of HIV is enough to do the trick (and that therefore one is therefore wanton and careless for having had sex in the first place).

As Vass (1986) has recently shown in his research, there was still in 1986 substantial credence for the idea that AIDS is attributable to homosexuality and promiscuity. While this attributes the problem to lifestyle, it also pays tribute to the consistency with which AIDS has been portrayed as an *illness of difference*. This continual articulation of difference and non-difference is a crucial part of the rhetoric of normalization that dominates media coverage of AIDS. In this respect, it is particularly informative to look at the recent television film *An Early Frost* and to consider the ways in which it depicted AIDS.

An Early Frost was the first television drama on the subject of AIDS to be seen nationwide in America, and inevitably the pressures of mass audience production have had an overwhelming influence on the quality of information and the range of representations within it. From the start, its producers, the National Broadcasting Company (NBC) were anxious lest they be seen to condone homosexuality, and because of this nervousness, the writers were forced to focus on the family's reaction to their son's illness. *An Early Frost* thus recruited AIDS for family drama, thereby exploring the stigma of the condition through the reactions of the family rather than through the personal problems that AIDS engenders. The film therefore works with a similar rhetoric and moral position to the early twentieth century American health propaganda films on venereal disease that Kuhn has analyzed (Kuhn, 1985). *An Early Frost* did not seek to provide a gay perspective on AIDS. Indeed, it was made by people who had very little knowledge of the subject matter before they embarked on the project. They were in a sense dealing with a social problem, both in order to feed a growing public disquiet about AIDS and to make it clear that NBC, just as much as any federal government agency, was prepared to tackle the problem of AIDS.

The producers of *An Early Frost* presumably identified their audience as overwhelmingly white, middle-class and suburban since the film admits little diversity of race, class and lifestyle, either in its depiction of gay men or of a family in shock. Instead, it establishes a set of oppositions — family versus faggots, living versus dying, father versus son which reinforce the message that AIDS is inevitably a source of conflict — something alien, a threat to normality.

Michael, played by Aidan Quinn, is a young lawyer, obviously successful and unaware that he is ill at the beginning of the film. By the end, he has been revealed to his family as a 'homosexual', and to us as a victim of AIDS and of his lover's promiscuous indiscretion. The decision was taken that Michael would not die in the course of the film; the period is covered is limited to the first two months after diagnosis. The NBC Vice-president in charge of the programme commented, 'there is a danger if we underrepresent the severity of the disease. But there is also the danger of overrepresenting it, if it is so graphic that it becomes too exploitative' (Farber, 1985). Of course, in one sense the public already know what people with AIDS look like. Stereotypically portrayed as wasted, and raddled with the blotches of Kaposi's sarcoma, they end up with drips and tubes pinning them down in hospital beds, their hands nothing but flesh and bone trailing across the sheets. They evoke pity, guilt and revulsion in much the same way as do people in Africa dying of hunger.

Images like these, which so clearly establish AIDS as something different, can be found in pictorial representations and in many articles in magazines. By and large they are inaccurate, offensive and deeply upsetting to those diagnosed as HIV antibody positive or with AIDS itself. But attempts to portray AIDS through bodily and social differences are not confined to the media portrayals of gay men with AIDS.

Simon Kinnersley is a journalist who has in his own words 'witnessed a great deal of heartache and suffering', but this has not stopped him writing articles in *Woman's Own* that spare none of the gory details about the sheer dreadfulness of AIDS, that paint pictures of debilitation and powerlessness, indignity and crass depersonalization. Baby Matthew Kazup's 'arms and legs are like matchsticks, so stiff they barely move. His skin is desperately pale and drawn. Sometimes Matthew gets such wild fevers he losses 10 per cent of his body weight in a night'. And so it goes on. Matthew's mother remarks that although she is not bitter against the homosexual community, 'They were consenting adults, they did have a choice' (Kinnersley, 1986).

The Individualization of Responsibility

In this section I would like to explore some of the processes by which recent portrayals of AIDS have served to *individualize* responsibility for the disease. Some of these processes have their origins in the claims of those who have been reported. Others are more deeply embedded in the structures and conventions that have governed media reporting of AIDS itself.

The confessional interview has become a popular way of talking about illness, and 'confessions' by people with AIDS have become widespread, particularly in gay publications, (but also in a more horrendous fashion in the popular press). Many of these have sought to establish connections between AIDS and states of mind for which personal responsibility can be taken. In *Eclipse*, the newsletter of the San Franciscan organization Shanti, there was recently a prime example of the connections that can be made between emotional and physical health within the context of AIDS (Eclipse, 1986). Christian Heran, a gay man in his fifties, describes how his low self-esteem and lack of emotional fulfilment are only now being remedied by intensive co-counselling. The sub-text of this and many similar interviews, chiefly in American publications, suggests that emotional alienation has its inevitable physical consequences. This message is unlikely to be helpful to those who do feel isolated, confused or devasted by the effects that AIDS has had on them and/or their friends. A greater premium is being placed on commitment than adventure in gay relationships at present, and the deepening sense of inadequacy and isolation felt by many people who, for whatever reason, have not formed enduring and fulfilling relationships in their lives, can be greatly exacerbated by these messages.

Yet a further source of impetus behind this individualization of responsibility with respect to AIDS has come from sections of the holistic health care movement. Whilst there is substantial literature detailing the usefulness of holistic therapy for the treatment of a wide variety of illness, less clearly articulated are the implications of holistic health care for AIDS itself. However, the books and articles which do exist present a somewhat contradictory set of claims with respect to the etiology of AIDS and the holistic health care interventions that might take place. There are some authors who have gone so far as to suggest that feelings of personal inadequacy and self-hate may actually 'cause' AIDS. Sally Fisher, founder of a New York project called *AIDS Mastery* has been quoted as saying,

> If we are angry enough with ourselves, then we may see our immune system reflect our deep feeling that we are unworthy of being protected. A friend suggested that AIDS is Anger Incorrectly Directed at the Self. (Fisher, 1986)

In a similar vein, the Neuro-Linguistic Programming therapist, Richard

Bandler, has suggested that illness can be looked at only by separating the body into different parts and functions. In order to understand why one has a disease, it is first necessary to ask the diseased part to come forward and enter into a dialogue. Only once someone has put themselves in the place of their diseased part can the reasons for their illness and the function that it performs for the body and psyche be understood and dealt with.

There are numerous other ideological currents that seek to individualize responsibility for health and illness which may also have a bearing on contemporary understandings of AIDS. Some of these have their origins in continuing debates about the relative responsibility of the individual and the state with respect to the provision of health care. Edwina Currie put it most succinctly at a recent conference in Newcastle when she declared that people's problems to do with health in the north-east of England are largely 'ignorance and (a) failing to realize that they do have some control over their lives' (*Guardian*, 1986). The idea of personal responsibility for health care has been repeatedly counterposed to the need for state intervention in this field in recent years (Homans and Aggleton's contribution to this book looks more closely at the idea of personal responsibility for health and the implications of this for styles of health education). In a country such as Britain where the state has come to control the health care services largely through a process of enlightened, concessionary liberalism, the health care services are inevitably subject to neo liberal ideologies and interventions such as those emanating from the present Conservative government, not only in terms of expenditure, but more importantly in terms of the ideological role which the National Health Service has to fulfil.

Currie later qualified her statement by saying that it was her aim to remind people that they do have some control over their health, that she wants to help people remain healthy rather than miss work, and that she wants women to have children 'that will remain healthy into manhood (sic)' (*Guardian*, 1986). Her concerns in this respect are telling. She is speaking almost for a nineteenth-century view of public health, one in which a healthy and reproductive populace is a wealthy and peaceable one. There is no room in pronouncements such as these for the marginal classes — those likely to include the groups first affected by AIDS. Her view of health education is normative and economistic, reflecting the ideological uses to which the National Health Service has been put by the present government. One does not have to look far beyond Currie's pronouncements for evidence of this. The present Conservative government has long vacillated over funding for screening for cervical cancer, for vaccination campaigns for those most at risk for Hepatitis B, and of course for AIDS research and treatment (although at the time of writing, limited funds had just been made available for cervical cancer and AIDS).

New Standards of Health?

So far, I have highlighted many of the dangers associated with the ways in which AIDS has come to be popularly represented. I have argued that metaphorically, AIDS has been identified as a *disease of difference*. I have also suggested that via a set of complex and contradictory processes, the origins of AIDS, both for the individual and for society at large, have simultaneously been linked to both *choice* and *destiny*. Finally, I have pointed to some of the disparate forces that seek to *individualize responsibility for health care intervention* within the context of AIDS. But events are rarely as uni-directional as this type of analysis would suggest, and in this final section I would like to consider some of the countervailing forces that may yet change our understanding of AIDS and the types of health care that are most suited to human needs.

In order to do this, I will return first to the nature of holistic health care intervention with respect to AIDS. I would like to begin by suggesting that the holistic health movement may yet have an important influence on attitudes towards health and illness by identifying new standards of health care. With a few exceptions (discussed above) holistic therapists by and large do not blame the patient for becoming ill. Despite a large number of books and articles which have suggested that people may become ill through 'character deficiencies' such as repressed anger, anxiety and inability to cope with stress (Savan, 1986), holistic practitioners do not believe that health is connected with character *per se*. For them, health is largely an issue of power, and it is the responsibility of the practitioner to show the patient how to reclaim power by which to take control of their lives in order to restore themselves to good health.

Within the context of AIDS, Christopher Spence (1986) for example has claimed that, 'by developing self-love, eliminating isolation from our lives, and making them at every level an impelling expression of the decision to refuse any limits on what is possible for each of us', we can flight illness and restore health (p. 9).

Powerlessness, weakness, defeat and death have long been part of the metaphorical construction of illness, yet they remain largely unchallenged within conventional medicine. Its practices, may pay lip service to the individuality of the person, but deprive most patients of any comprehensive understanding of their illness, their prognosis and their treatment.

Breast cancer provides a good example of the way in which women are expected to follow medical advice without knowing how contentious all medical knowledge is in this area. Jo Spence, whose photographic study *A Picture of Health* examines alternative approaches to breast cancer, has now abandoned conventional treatment and is following a variety of naturopathic treatments chosen by herself. Although the cancer initially recurred on the mastectomy site, Spence now feels that the tumour is under control and will continue to diminish while she remains in full control of her treatment, refusing all chemotherapy (Spence, 1986a and 1986b).

Writers such as Jo Spence advocate the greater availability of holistic treatment, and more importantly, the beginning of a dialogue between holistic practice and conventional medicine; not necessarily in order to change medical theory but in order for patients to gain greater control over their treatment as doctors come to more widely accept the benefits which greater patient responsibility can bring. In this respect, the various consequences of HIV infection may occupy a crucial position in changing discourses to do with health and power. Whilst medical understanding of these consequences develops daily, the question is not often asked — who decides in which direction the research around AIDS should proceed?

Allopathic therapies for AIDS remain the main symbol of hope for many people despite the evidence to date that one drug alone is unlikely to cure the disease. Research remains stubbornly directed towards a relatively small number of areas that might prove beneficial in widespread treatment. By and large, researchers have so far ignored the claims of holistic medicine to offer a better understanding of the illness, in particular of the effects of diet on the immune system, and of the way in which the body might work to heal itself (as well as how drugs might interfere with this process).

The politics of medical research have been undoubtedly influential in framing our understanding of HIV infection and AIDS, and we must not ignore the extent to which medicine itself uses metaphorical understandings of illness to sustain its own economy and practices. Cancer and AIDS have both been 'attacked' and had war waged on them; being 'enemies' to be defeated through the use of chemical, nuclear and conventional forces in a struggle for the survival of civilization. In a sense, they are both Cold War diseases. The fight against cancer began in the 1950s as other infectious diseases became less deadly — its epidemiology and treatment thus became susceptible to the newly enlivened metaphors. Since then, it has to some extent been sold to the American taxpayer as part of the defence budget — a problem to be defeated by new and wonderful 'weapons' along with world communism. Whether, during this escalation of conflict, the US government will decide to initiate a Star Wars type programme to deal with AIDS remains to be seen.

Drug companies obviously need epidemics; they need identifiable scourges to vanquish, and they need the Federal Food and Drug Administration (FFDA) to police their activities in order to maintain public confidence in their position within the health economy. An American New Right columnist recently suggested that a cure for AIDS would be found if only the FFDA were to stop regulating standards so strictly. In reality, the drug companies need the federal attention to new diseases, markets and cures in order to sustain a rationalized programme of research, development, production and profit. Yet should AIDS be recruited to enliven the free market, we may find that the metaphorical links between social order and the nature of illness are not only stronger than might be imagined, but marvellously supple too!

As yet there has been little pressure from outside the medical profession over the direction of research. This appears to be due to a widespread ignorance both about the ways in which the goals of research are determined, and about the range of possibilities for research that exist with respect to HIV infection. If people with AIDS and others are to demand a widening of research being carried out in relation to HIV infection, then they must first promote widespread discussion of what is presently understood about the disease amongst those at risk as well as engage in public dialogue with doctors and scientists. To do otherwise, is to reinforce widespread acceptance of the view that 'doctors know best', thus denying those with HIV infection the opportunity to take control of their treatment.

HIV infection has also challenged established medical practice in other ways, notably with respect to the care of the terminally ill and the etiquette of diagnosis. *The Lighthouse*, a community support centre in London, was designed in the words of Christopher Spence (1986), for 'guiding people safely home' (p. 65), by providing an environment where people with HIV infection can find support at various stages in their illness. It is neither a hospice nor a social centre, but is intended to integrate the many forms of support and counselling required by those with HIV infection without dividing people into the categories, HIV antibody positive, AIDS Related Complex (ARC), AIDS and dying, thereby showing that health is a continuum.

Organizations such as Body Positive and the Terrence Higgins Trust in Britain have also managed to persuade some larger hospitals of the necessity for post-diagnosis support and counselling — something which is relatively unheard of with respect to other forms of illness. Body Positive has also begun to challenge power relations within mainstream medical practice in other ways, being not only a support group for people who have been diagnosed as HIV antibody positive, but also a crucial source of information and advice that is not mediated by the medical profession. Similar organizations exist on a smaller scale for other illnesses, but as HIV infection becomes more prevalent, it is possible that Body Positive will assume an increasingly important role in campaigns for patient-centred care in an illness that has such a high profile.

Thus we have a situation in which self-help and community-oriented activity around AIDS has a positive contribution to make not only to our understanding of human immune function, but also to the rights of patients and the nature of health care more generally. It will be instructive to observe the extent to which the medical profession as a whole embraces the changes that intervention with respect to HIV infection may demand, and how in turn this may affect health care practice in the future.

References

AMIS, M. (1985) 'Making sense out of AIDS', *The Observer*, 23 June.

BLAND, L. and MORT, E. (1983) 'Look out for the good time girl', *Formations of Nation and People*, London, Routledge and Kegan Paul.

DOYAL, L. with PENNELL, I. (1979) *The Political Economy of Health*, London, Pluto Press.

Eclipse (1986) Spring Newsletter.

FARBER, S. (1985) 'Family loyalty', *New York Times*.

FISHER, S. (1986) 'Consider the alternative', *Village Voice*, 27 May.

FOUCAULT, M. (1973) *The Birth of the Clinic*, London, Tavistock

FOUCAULT, M. (1979) *The History of Sexuality*. Volume 1, Harmondsworth, Penguin Books.

GOLDSTEIN, R. (1983) 'Heartsick; Fear and loving in the gay community', *Village Voice*, 28 June.

Guardian (1986) Report on Speech by Edwina Currie, 24 September .

KINNERSLEY, S. (1986) 'Your baby's got AIDS', *Woman's Own*. 3 May.

KUHN, A. (1985) *The Power of the Image*: *Essays on Representations and Sexuality*. London, Routledge and Kegan Paul.

MCGRATH, R. (1984) 'The medical police', *Ten/8*, 14.

PATTON, C. (1985) *Sex and Germs*: *The Politics of AIDS*. Boston, MA, South End Press.

SAVAN, L. (1986) 'Consider the alternative', *Village Voice*. 27 May.

SONTAG, S. (1983) *Illness as Metaphor*, Hardmondsworth, Penguin Books.

SPENCE, C. (1986) *AIDS: Time to Reclaim our Power*. London, Lifestory.

SPENCE, J. (1986a) 'Body beautiful or body in crisis?', *Open Mind*, June/July.
SPENCE, J. (1986b) 'The picture of health', *Spare Rib*, 163. pp. 19–24.
VASS, A. (1986) *A Plague in Us*. Cambridge, Venus Academica.
WEEKS, J. (1985) *Sexuality and its Discontents*, London, Routledge and Kegan
    Paul.

5
Perceptions of risk — Media treatment of AIDS

Kaye Wellings

The mass media is increasingly recognized by those concerned with educating the public as offering an extremely effective channel for communicating health messages. It provides the possibility of reaching more people, including those who might not otherwise be contacted, and it allows for a more sophisticated presentation of material than do many more formal educational processes.

However, health educators have not always paid sufficient attention to the ways in which the media might misinform the public by distorting medical and scientific findings, by paying selective attention to particular types of evidence compared with others, or by simply getting it wrong.

In this sense, media reporting of AIDS offers us a good case study of the ways in which the mass media can do health education a disservice. As Altman (1986) has pointed out, AIDS has gained an unprecedented amount of media attention for two main reasons — first, because AIDS has proved to be near inevitably fatal, and second, because in the popular imagination it has been associated with forms of sexual behaviour which have provided opportunities for sensationalist and voyeuristic reporting.

Because people's behavioural responses are based very much upon their perceptions of risk, much of the work of health educators is crucially concerned with helping their clients assess risks; to balance, contain or reduce them. The ways in which people perceive risk within the context of a disease such as AIDS will, however, be influenced by their conceptualization of certain key aspects of the syndrome. In particular, they will be associated with who is most perceived to be affected, what the causes are, how many are affected and how the disease is transmitted. My aim in this chapter is to look at some of the ways in which one section of the mass media — national newspaper journalism — reported on these aspects of AIDS early in the epidemic between 1983 and 1985, and to contrast this with what might be seen as the 'official' information about the syndrome that was concurrently put out by health educators. In the process of doing this, I will try to identify certain discontinuities and contradictions which have serious implications for popular judgments of risk.

Who Is Affected?

A Gay Plague?

Before the Equality Council of the National Union of Journalists (NUJ) issued guidance on the reporting of AIDS in 1984 (and in more than a few instances, well after this) AIDS was virtually synonymous with the term 'gay plague' in national press reportage in Britain. This description was used as often in the 'quality' press ('"gay plague" may lead to blood ban on homosexuals', *Daily Telegraph*, 2 May 1983; 'gay plague sets off panic', *Observer*, 26 June 1983) as it was in the tabloids ('watchdogs in "gay plague" blood probe', *Sun*, 2 May 1983; 'alert over "gay plague"', *Daily Mirror*, 2 May 1983). Even where cases of the disease were reported in the context of other 'high risk' groups, the widespread use of this term has meant that AIDS has come to be perceived as a disease afflicting mainly homosexual men.

Since the NUJ's action in 1984, AIDS has continued to be portrayed as a predominantly homosexual disease, in spite of gradually emerging evidence of its prevalence within heterosexual populations. Evidence suggesting that the origins of the disease may have been other than within the homosexual community have tended to be censored in many cases and where cases of the disease occurring in other groups have been identified, a rather different style of reporting has been adopted.

Although there is some statistical basis for the claim that AIDS is a disease affecting mainly gay men in the West, (about nine out of ten cases so far have involved homosexual men in the UK, and about seven out of ten in the US), this has not been the case worldwide. As early as the middle of 1983, reports began to be published which gave grounds for considering that AIDS might have originated, not in New York, San Francisco or Haiti, but in Central Africa where the sex ratio for those affected by the disease was strongly suggestive of heterosexual transmission, and where cases did not fall into the 'risk groups' characteristic of the West (Clumeck *et al*, 1983). In November 1983 at a meeting on AIDS at the World Health Organization in Geneva new evidence from Central

Africa and the Caribbean was presented which suggested that AIDS could be transmitted via routine sexual contact between women and men (*New Scientist*, 1983).

The 'African Connection'

By the middle of 1984 there was a lively debate in British medical journals concerning whether AIDS was a 'new' disease or an 'old' disease endemic in Central Africa which had perhaps gone unrecognized because of imprecise diagnosis, and which had somehow found a new susceptible host in the West.[1] As this debate got under way, two important differences emerged between the African cases of AIDS and those in Europe and North America. First, there was a completely different sex distribution. In Zaire, for example, the ratio of men to women with AIDS was eleven to ten (compared with fifteen to one in Europe at that time). Second, African cases did not appear to fall into what, in Europe and North America, were now recognized as particular 'risk groups' (homosexual/bisexual men, injecting drug users etc).

This evidence challenged the widely held belief at the time that AIDS had originated in Haiti and had travelled to America via gay men returning from vacation there, and thence to Europe. Instead, it was now suggested that Haitians working in Africa shortly after independence had taken back with them an originally heterosexual disease which had then spread to the population of gay American holidaymakers in Haiti. This debate over whether AIDS originated in Haiti or Central Africa is, of course, somewhat reminiscent of earlier sixteenth century arguments about whether syphilis was a 'French' or an 'Italian' disease (Felstein, 1974). Nevertheless, the 'African connection', threw into serious doubt prior theories concerning the homosexual origins of AIDS and seemed at least as plausible as rival accounts.

This 'African connection' was reported fairly widely in the non tabloid press. In an early report in the *Sunday Times* (11 March 1984), for example, it was claimed that, 'The disease almost certainly came to this country from the United States; but it appears to have originated in Central Africa'. Later in the same year, the *Guardian* (31 October 1984) carried a long feature under the headline 'The AIDS that Africa could do without'. The article began by claiming that, 'Retrospective analysis shows that AIDS has been present in Zaire since at least 1976', and ended on the note, 'Homosexuals have always objected to AIDS being called the gay plague. The evidence now shows they are right'.

Not until 1985, however, were the possible heterosexual and African origins of AIDS mentioned by the tabloid press. Initially only one newspaper, the *Daily Mirror* (5 March 1985), took the story up and paradoxically, even in this context, AIDS was still referred to the 'gay plague' — 'AIDS is believed to have struck first in Africa and spread rapidly ... from Africa, the disease leapt the Atlantic to the Caribbean and then to the United States. Infected Americans brought it to England and Europe and now the 'gay plague' has spread right around the world to Australia'.

Innocent Victims and Guilty Agents

Journalists have tended to adopt very different styles of reporting, both quantitatively and qualitatively, depending on whether those who contracted the disease are homosexual or heterosexual. Although from early on in the epidemic, AIDS has been depicted as a 'gay plague', the deaths of individual gay men from the disease were usually only summarily mentioned, perhaps in an odd column inch or so of newspaper space and often simply by number — '37th AIDS death' (*Daily Telegraph*, 17 February 1984); '39th AIDS death' (*Sun*, 5 December 1984). In contrast, the deaths of heterosexuals outside the 'high risk' groups were prominently and extensively featured. The first death of a baby from AIDS in Britain, for example, was allotted the whole of the front page of the *Daily Mail* (12 May 1985) and was given prominent coverage in all the daily nationals.

Admittedly, what is newsworthy tends to be the exception rather than the rule, and where cases of AIDS amongst gay men offered interesting contradictions they did receive more attention. A great deal has been made journalistically, for example, of cases involving men of the Church, but in these instances only veiled reference is usually made to the possible sexual orientation of those involved. An article 'AIDS kills Church of England curate', for example, featured in the *Daily Mail* (28 June 1984) stated, 'The death of 31-year-old Father Ian Robson from the illness nicknamed "the gay plague", because most of its victims are homosexuals, has shaken the church establishment ... Father Robson, who was *unmarried* ...'. In the same newspaper (1 February 1985) a prison chaplain who died from AIDS was described somewhat coyly as 'The Rev Gregory Edwards, a 38-year-old *bachelor* ...' (emphasis added in both cases).

Understandably perhaps, anonymity has sometimes resulted from the ruling of coroners that the names of gay men who have died subsequent to

AIDS should not be disclosed in order to safeguard the possible sensitivities of families and friends. But generally speaking, the fleshing out of personal biographies in a way that would allow readers to empathize with those concerned has been far more common in relation to cases of AIDS involving non-homosexuals. In particular, the human faces put to the clinical cases have tended to be those of heterosexuals who have inadvertently caught the disease via a route which was other than sexual. Thus haemophiliacs and the recipients of blood transfusions have been singled out for sympathetic attention from the media as have children and the elderly.

There is further evidence that journalists and editors have often selected cases with which it has been thought the public might most easily identify. A journalist who approached Dr Anthony Pinching of St Mary's Hospital, London, in search of a story reputedly said that he 'couldn't run a story about gay men because his readers weren't interested — what they were interested in was blood'.[2]

Newspaper reporting on AIDS has thereby tended to differentiate between so-called 'innocent' and 'guilty' victims of the syndrome. On the whole, the deaths of those who have contracted the disease as a result of what some may see as 'illicit' or 'morally unacceptable' practices (by being gay, by being bisexual, by being a prostitute or by being an intravenous drug user) have been evaluated far more negatively by the media than those of people who have become infected as a result of accidental or iatrogenic infection (through blood transfusions or through the use of contaminated blood products). Those falling into this latter category have often been depicted as the 'innocent victims' of disease in much the same way as civilian casualties are often reported by war correspondents. In a headline story involving a schoolchild with AIDS, for example, the *Daily Express* (25 September 1985) asked, 'AIDS: Why must the innocent suffer?' and Mary Kenny commented in the *Sunday Telegraph* (3 February 1985), 'Of course people should not be persecuted or blamed for catching AIDS, because that is vindictive and uncharitable and anyway, it *can* be caught *innocently*' (emphasis added). At the same time, headlines like that in the *Daily Telegraph* (20 May 1983) 'Alarm as lethal "plague" spreads to non-homosexuals' have helped reinforce the dangerous idea that there has been a 'leakage' of infection from a culpable minority to a blame-free population.

The suggestion that some people with AIDS (PWAs) might actually 'deserve' the disease has generated some ambivalent attitudes towards research into a cure or vaccine. For example, when Alter *et al* (1984) in *Science* magazine reported on a study to determine whether chimpanzees might provide an animal model for AIDS in the context of developing a vaccine, the *Sunday Mirror* (4 December 1983) described the study under the headline 'Torture of innocents: Chimps in "sex plague" tests'. Its account continued,

> Healthy chimpanzees are being injected with the mystery killer disease AIDS in a new bid to find a cure for humans. The condition — Acquired Immune Deficiency Syndrome — is known as the 'gay plague' because it mainly affects homosexuals. Animal-lovers are horrified. They have started massive campaigns to stop the research which could lead to a horrible and lingering death for the animals.

A very different style of reporting has been adopted to describe the plight of those deemed to be the 'guilty victims' of infection. Here, there is rarely any attempt to elicit the compassion of readers. PWAs in this category are often rendered faceless and depersonalized so that it was difficult to sympathize with them. Where personal accounts have been provided, they have often been written in such a way as to incite horror and repugnance in the reader. In both the *News of the World* (6 January 1985) and the *Sunday People* (24 July 1983) photographs showing the once handsome faces of young gay men have been juxtaposed against those ravaged by the progressive toll of the disease.

Compassion on the other hand has tended to be reserved for non-homosexual sufferers, and is usually called for in wildly emotive language. The plight of a haemophiliac PWA, for example, was described in the *Daily Mail* (20 November 1984) under the headline 'Seven-month *hell* of man dying from AIDS'; and a baby who contracted AIDS was described as a '*heartbreak* baby' by the *Sun* (10 November 1983) (both with emphasis added).

Moral Ambiguity and the Reporting of AIDS

What the print media has seemed less inclined to report on are cases of AIDS more marginal to the moral categories than these two groups. Cases of heterosexual transmission where there is no evidence of unorthodox or illicit sexual practices have rarely been reported. Similarly, cases which do not fit easily into the stereotypes so far identified have either been ignored or re-conceptualized editorially. Amazingly, the death of the first women in Britain as a result of AIDS acquired through heterosexual intercourse (Smith *et al*, 1983) passed virtually unreported by the national press.

Another example of censoring out of cases of the disease involving 'normal' heterosexual transmission is again provided by Dr A Pinching.[2] In February 1985, the British Medical Journal reported the case of a 50-year-old married woman who had had *one* sexual partner and who had contracted gonorrhea and AIDS three and a half years after divorcing him. After first checking with the patient to see whether she would be willing to disclose the details of the case to the press, Dr Pinching tried to interest a journalist in the case. But although the case was described in local newspapers at the time (*Sunday Advertiser*, 22 February 1985; *Evening Echo*, 22 February 1985), none of the nationals were willing to pick it up.

A striking example of the way in which the media has attempted to 'edit' PWAs into appropriate moral categories can be found in a report by Rose *et al* (1983) reported in the *Lancet*. This concerns a Canadian nun who had been working with prostitutes in Haiti. The original report stressed that the woman had only one male sexual contact and that 'no other risk factor except residence in Haiti was present'. This was fairly accurately reported in articles in the *Daily Telegraph*, the *Daily Mirror* and the *Sun* (17 September 1983), all of which stressed the link with Haiti. But editorially the stories in the *Daily Telegraph* and the *Sun* were headlined as, 'Vice work nun dies of AIDS' and 'Gay plague kills isle's red light nun' respectively. Thus, by association the nun is magically transported epidemiologically from the Haitian 'risk group' linked more closely with illicit sex.

The human faces given to PWAs then have by and large been those of heterosexuals infected by the virus through routes other than sexual transmission. Moral categories based on distinctions between such qualities as innocent/guilty and undeserving/deserving have hereby been overlain like a template onto the various clinically defined 'risk groups'. Where cases of AIDS have occurred which are marginal to these differently evaluated 'risk groups'; where they have fallen between categories, and where the moral categories have not been consonant with the medical ones, the tendency has been for the cases to be 'edited' to fit existing categories. Alternatively they have simply been omitted altogether from popular press reports. In consequence, heterosexual transmission of HIV between women and men has been rendered largely invisible and hidden from view.

This polarization of PWAs into the 'innocent' and the 'guilty', and the perceived exclusivity of the disease in terms of those affected, has had a powerful effect on public perceptions of who is at risk. A pervasive feeling that only those who 'deserve' AIDS will fall prey to infection has encouraged the lay belief that the syndrome is a 'curse of the other' — a disease which single-mindedly selects those deserving of misfortune. Moreover, as we have seen, mass media reporting of AIDS (in newspapers at least) has tended to focus on 'at risk' *groups* rather than on 'at risk' *behaviours* and *sexual practices*. Given what we currently know about the ways in which HIV can be transmitted, in health educational terms it would be better to talk in terms of the behaviours which facilitate viral transmission rather than the supposed pre-disposition of groups to infection. The crucial variable determining whether or not an individual will become infected by the virus is after all not their *identity* or their membership of a particular *group*, but sexual or blood contact with an already infected person.

What Causes AIDS?

Until the discovery in late 1983 of an AIDS-associated virus, the fact that AIDS principally affected gay men (in Europe and North America at least) had prompted researchers to look for some distinctive features relating to male homosexual behaviour in their search for a cause. Initially attention was focussed on aspects of the 'gay lifestyle' itself — on 'fast lane' living; frequent sex with multiple partners, late hours, inadequate nourishment and regular drug taking, including the use of sexually stimulating drugs. Before the isolation of HIV as a viral agent, the claim that life-style was associated with AIDS was not linked to the argument that the sexual behaviour of gay men might simply increase the probability of being exposed to a particular pathogen. Rather, it was identified as a direct causal factor. For example, Lacey and Waugh (1983) writing in the *Lancet* (20 August 1983) claimed that, 'There are some theoretical grounds for believing that the nature of homosexual coitus can cause immunosuppression.'

Although these life-style theories of causation were multifactorial in their emphasis, they tended to collapse the distinction between psychosocial, environmental and biological factors. The sexual behaviour of gay men came thereby to be seen not so much as a *facilitator* of disease transmission as an organic *cause* of it. Several theories developed along these lines and were reported at the time in the medical journals. Some writers suggested that semen itself might weaken the body's immune system, speculating that men were immunologically less well equipped than women to deal with it, particularly when large amounts were absorbed orally and anally (Hsia *et al*, 1984). Others have presented dubious and controversial evidence implicating the use of sexual stimulants such as amyl and butyl nitrite ('poppers') in the impairment of the body's immune system (Jorgensen, 1982; Marmor *et al*, 1982; Goedert *et al*, 1982).

One particular theory which gained widespread acceptance in the early days was that of 'immune overload'. This suggested that the repeated onslaught of sexually transmitted infections and the regular use of antibiotics might cause an already-compromised immune system to undergo total break down (see for example, Marmor *et al*, 1982; Gyorkey *et al*, 1982; Oswald *et al*, 1982). According to Waterson (1983), 'the ... sheer weight of chemical and microbial insult to the body in general, and to T-lymphocytes in particular, goes beyond the tolerable limit. Eventually irreparable damage is sustained, which becomes manifest clinically in one or other of the variety of components of the syndrome.'

Even at the time, 'immune overload' theories had little epidemiological or clinical plausibility. Nitrites had been in medicinal use for the treatment of angina for a number of decades and no systematic effects on the immune system had been identified. Cytomegaloviral infection (one of the sexually transmitted infections most implicated in early versions of 'immune overload' theory) is present in most adults without serious complication. And there is little evidence that the human immune system simply wears out or collapses under pressure. Besides which, AIDS is not confined epidemiologically to individuals with prior multiple infections nor to those who have used 'poppers'. But the major problem with 'immune overload' theories was that they failed to explain infectivity. If AIDS was caused by a 'lifestyle' or behaviour alone, it would be unlikely to be a communicable disease, and epidemiological evidence strongly suggested the contrary in this respect.

Several writers in the medical journals recognized these flaws and hedged their bets by identifying lifestyle factors as one factor contributing to the etiology of the syndrome alongside other, possibly viral, causes. When a viral agent was eventually identified as a possible cause of AIDS (speculatively in middle to late 1983, and more confidently in 1984), the major defect associated with 'immune overload' theories was acknowledged. In terms of immuno-suppression, such explanations had put the cart before the horse. Immune deficiency was not the *cause* of AIDS, but its *consequence*.

As a result, 'immune overload' theories largely lost their credibility and more or less disappeared from the medical literature. But in the lay press they have lingered on in one form or another, both implicitly in continued reference to the link between 'gay lifestyles' and AIDS, and occasionally in even more explicit forms. For example, in an article in the

Observer (23 June 1985) somewhat inappropriately titled 'Making sense of AIDS', it was claimed that,

> Throughout the past decade, in New York, gay men were oppressed by an escalating series of health hazards. To begin with, crabs, gonorrhoea and syphilis, the ancient enemies. Then herpes, then cytomegalovirus, then gay bowel syndrome, then hepatitis B. All venereal diseases compromise the immune system. And so, crucially, does semen. Semen contains antigens, foreign elements which stimulate the production of antibodies. The female body has ways of deactivating semen; the male body has no such strategies. At each reception the immune system goes on red alert. Ironically, it too becomes paranoid. Repeated infection and repeated *trauma* prolong the crisis until the cells lose the capacity to correct their own over-correction.

The identification of a specific pathogen as a cause of AIDS did not eliminate this opportunity to attach blame to selected groups of those who fell prey to the disease. In media reports, the virus was not seen to strike randomly, but rather to purposefully single out certain groups on the basis of their gender and their sexual orientation. In this same article in the *Observer*, the author went on to write,

> If the AIDS virus had chosen, say, real-estate agents or young mothers for attack, then the medical and social context would now look very different. Yet AIDS has *chosen* homosexual men. (emphasis added)

There is more than a hint of intentionality here, something which has been common in other press reports which imply that gay men have offended against a supposedly 'natural' order, and in consequence the virus has been sent by vengeful nature or a retributive God to punish them. In the *Sunday Express* (24 February 1985), John Junor has written, 'If AIDS is not an Act of God with consequences just as frightful as fire and brimstone, then just what the hell is it?' and in a similar but more elliptical vein a leader in *The Times* (3 November 1984) has claimed, 'Many members of the public are tempted to see in AIDS some sort of retribution for a questionable life style, but AIDS of course is a danger not only to the promiscuous nor only to homosexuals'.

Some commentators went further than this to suggest that AIDS may be a disease whose mysteries may never be understood, by medical science or otherwise. Instead, they are best left as a matter for divine wisdom.

Manifestly the health authorities are baffled, and it is no good homosexuals expecting much from them, at any rate in the foreseeable future. Yet such pronouncements as there are all come from doctors and medical officers, etc. Is it not time that the bishops brought God into the act, since one suspects that religious fanatics — condemned by homosexuals as ignorant bigots — who talk about the wrath of God may know more about the cause of the disease, and its cure, than at present do all the scientists working together. (Peregrine Worsthorne, *Sunday Telegraph*, 10 February 1985)

These are of course extreme, but by no means isolated, examples of the tone of some modern reporting. Other writers, recognizing perhaps that such views may not gain much popularity in a largely secular society, have used reported speech and allusion to the views of third parties to make similar references. The *Sun* (7 February 1985) for example has carried the headline 'AIDS is the wrath of God, says vicar' and the *Daily Telegraph* (3 May 1983) has used quotation marks to create a similar effect '"Wages of sin" A deadly toll'.

How Many People are Affected?

It is difficult to exaggerate the seriousness of AIDS: a fatal disease which affects people in their prime and for which there is neither a vaccine nor a cure does not need to be particularly widespread in order to warrant concern. Moreover, because of the disease's long incubation period, together with uncertainty about how many of those infected will eventually develop it, estimates of prevalence based on currently observable incidence provide little reliable indication of the potential reservoir of infection in the population as a whole.

Nevertheless, widespread statistical distortions have occurred in the press coverage which are not simply a function of uncertainty within the data. Before the isolation and identification of HIV, prevalence was estimated by examining selected populations for markers which might indicate the presence of infection. Reports of such studies in the medical journals were often hedged with reservations about the data, and cautioned against attaching too much importance to the predictive value of findings from relatively small-scale studies of specific sub-groups — usually gay men routinely attending clinics for the treatment of sexually transmitted diseases (STD clinics).

In spite of this, newspaper reports often wildly extrapolated from this clinical data to the wider population, with scant regard for base rates or the caveats of the original authors. A study of cellular immunity amongst gay men attending the STD clinic at St Mary's Hospital, London, for example, showed that 12 per cent of symptom-free clinic attenders had lymphocyte abnormalities characteristic of AIDS and 5 per cent also had anergy, the index combination of defects seen in AIDS (Pinching *et al*, 1983). This study was reported in the *Observer* (7 August 1983). The text of the article began, '*Thousands* of gay men in Britain may already have the abnormalities of the immune system associated with the killer disease AIDS' (emphasis added). The qualifying 'may' in the text was dropped in the headline accompanying the report which simply read, 'Thousands of British gays have symptoms of AIDS'. Headlines of course make the initial impact on the reader and again it was here, at the editorial level, that any sense of equivocation was lost. In the text of the article itself, however, little attempt was made to explain that many of the signs described are common to people who do not have AIDS. Still less was it suggested that findings from a central London STD clinic may not be generalizable to the rest of the population. NUJ guidelines concerning the reporting of AIDS have drawn specific attention to this latter point.

Subsequent to the identification of an AIDS-associated virus and the development of tests for antibodies to this virus, there has been more opportunity to conduct prevalence studies. Research carried out by workers at the Public Health Laboratory Services in Colindale in 1985 suggested that 30 per cent of gay men tested in London and 5 per cent outside the capital could at that time be HIV antibody positive (Mortimer *et al*, 1985). Corresponding figures from the STD clinic at London's Middlesex Hospital suggested that in early 1985 upwards of 20 per cent of gay men attending the clinic were HIV antibody positive, and equivalent figures from St Mary's Hospital, London released at about the same time suggested that about 15 per cent of clinic attenders may have been infected.

Again, these findings were widely reported by the press with no reference to their denominators. *The Times* (19 April 1985) for example reported that, 'More than a third of tested homosexuals "showed evidence of the AIDS virus"', with no clear indication as to whether its claim referred to the total gay population, that of London or, as was the case here, gay men attending one London STD clinic. The *Daily Star* (4 February 1985) ran the headline 'AIDS threat to one in five: Gays are warned' and the *Daily Express* (8 February 1985) covered the same story with the claim that '15 per cent of gays in London are "infected"'.

Forecasts of the future incidence of AIDS have regularly been made by projecting forwards current rates of increase on the assumption that these will be sustained. In May 1984, the Royal College of Nursing, by a simple mathematical calculation, predicted that if numbers continued to double every six months, there would be a million cases of AIDS worldwide by the end of the century. Only *The Times* (4 May 1984) reported this claim, under the headline '"AIDS cases may reach a million" health chief says'. Interestingly, in the text of the accompanying article describing this dramatic prediction, the disease is called, in a stunning Freudian slip, 'AIDS, Acquired *Immoral* Deficiency Syndrome' (emphasis added).

By early 1985, three years after official recording of AIDS cases by the Communicable Diseases Surveillance Centre commenced, it was theoretically possible to carry out the exercise again with more reliable parameter estimates. In consequence, the Royal College of Nursing issued a second prediction of one million cases in Britain by 1991. This was reported verbatim or expressed as a rate of one in fifty by *The Times*, the *Sun*, the *Daily Mirror*, the *Daily Express* and the *Daily Star* (10 January 1985). The disparity between these two sets of figures — on the one hand a million cases worldwide within sixteen years, and on the other, the same number in Britain within only six years — must have led to a great deal of confusion in the public mind.

The medical and scientific press at the time, however, carried a discussion of the limitations of such exercises. Annual increases to date had been roughly exponential and therefore, if expressed *on a logarithmic scale*, plotted points were very close to a straight line. The obvious temptation was therefore to assume that this rate of increase would be sustained in future years. But as McEvoy and Tillett (1985) pointed out, for such predictions to be valid it would have to be assumed that all factors influencing the course of the epidemic would remain constant, that the numbers of most susceptible people would not drop, and that there would be no substantial changes in behaviour limiting the spread of infection. McEvoy and Tillett suggested that according to conventional statistical analysis, the 'real' figure in 1990 could (as estimated in 1985) turn out to be either as low as one case or as high as 295 million cases, within the same confidence limits. They warned that statistical predictions of future trends in the epidemic were not currently very useful.

The figures produced by the Royal College of Nursing were also challenged by the then Minister of Health who in the *Daily Express* (11 January 1985) accused the College of 'fancy maths'. But despite these various disclaimers, the potency of the one million figure made a deep impression on the public mind. Although some of these estimates, the worldwide one for example, may turn out to have some foundation, the British figure of one million by 1991 has already had to be revised downwards. Nevertheless, the scale on which AIDS was *apparently* spreading throughout the population made medical claims about the low infectivity of the disease seem strikingly implausible. Media messages suggesting the widespread prevalence of AIDS contrasted sharply with the claims of mainstream health education campaigns. The Health Education Council's booklet 'Some facts about AIDS' published in February 1985, for example, described the disease as 'a *rare condition* which prevents the body's defences from working properly' (emphasis added).

This confusion in the public mind was compounded by conflicting messages reported as coming from the government level. The need to generate public concern about AIDS within the context of health promotion, together with the need to quell the panic which had started to threaten social and medical services, made it difficult to put across a coherent and unified message. At the same time, uncertainty within the data on which future predictions were based made it possible for varying interpretations to be given to these. High expected prevalence figures were often used to alert people to the dangers of HIV infection, whereas lower figures relating the actual reported cases of AIDS were used to quieten the alarm. In a plea to members of the gay community to act to halt the spread of HIV infection, the Chief Medical Officer for England was quoted as predicting 5000 cases of AIDS in Britain within three years ('Medical chief tells gays how to avoid AIDS', *Sunday Times*, 10 February 1985). Whilst in a parallel attempt to provide reassurance to those working in the emergency services reported in the *Daily Telegraph* (19 February 1985) under the headline 'Don't halt kiss-of-life plea as fear of AIDS risk grows', he reportedly spoke of AIDS as a 'rare disease' with 'exaggerated risks'.

How Is the Disease Transmitted?

Possibly more myths and misunderstandings have surrounded the question of how HIV infection is passed from one person to another than any other single aspect of the disease. We now know that HIV is transmitted primarily, and it may turn out to be exclusively, through intimate sexual contact with, or via the blood of, an infected person. Yet as those who have answered enquiries from or given advice to the public are all too aware, misinformation is still rife. Whatever opinion polls may show people's rational responses to be, large sections of the population are still worried by insect bites, shared cups and cutlery, swimming pools, kissing and shaking hands as possible sources of infection.

Why have these myths persisted when so many efforts have been made to deal with them? To answer this question, we need to know far more about lay conceptions of illness in relation to AIDS. But we can also look to newspaper accounts for evidence of the ways in which these lay beliefs may have been reinforced or affirmed.

In fairness, most newspapers have been at pains to present often lengthy and detailed features identifying the main routes by which HIV can be transmitted, at the same time as they have pointed out that everyday contact with an infected person poses no risk of infection. Regular health education articles have been featured in some newspapers and medical experts have been called upon to write them. What we need to look at, however, is how well such accounts stand up against concurrent reporting of scare stories about AIDS which, repeatedly and consistently, undermine the impact of this more reliable information.

The major wave of media hype and public panic which began in early 1985, fuelled by fears of widespread transmission, has its origins in an article published in *Science* magazine with the title 'HTLV-III in saliva of people with AIDS-related complex and healthy homosexual men at risk for AIDS' (Groopman *et al*, 1984). This report revealed that HIV (called HTLV-III at that time) had been isolated in the laboratory, and with difficulty, from the saliva of some of those infected.

With a degree of prescience, an earlier article in the *Observer* (14 October 1984) had anticipated possible reactions to such a claim. Under the headline 'AIDS vendetta looms', the author wrote, ' .. it raises the prospect of a public vendetta against those who may be accused of passing on the disease in restaurants, offices, drinking fountains and other public places'. Later in the text, a biochemist is quoted as saying 'If saliva was the main way to transmit AIDS, we would be seeing hundreds of thousands of cases by now'.

The rest of the British press were slow to report this startling finding. Not until early the following year, and then initially only in the *News of the World* (20 January 1985) was it mentioned, under the headline 'Kiss of death' — 'Scientists now fear that the killer sex disease AIDS could be caught by just kissing. They have found traces of the dreaded virus in the saliva of victims'. However, the possibility of transmission via saliva was eventually to trigger a veritable flood of panic stories in the ensuing weeks (figure 1).

Subsequently, the press carried stories of gay men banned from work and barred from pubs and clubs — 'Club bans two gays in AIDS panic...

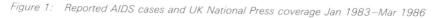

Figure 1:   Reported AIDS cases and UK National Press coverage Jan 1983–Mar 1986

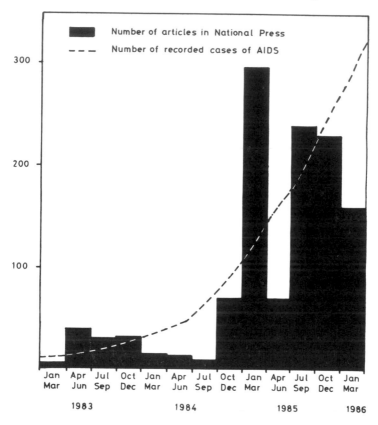

Beer mugs may spread disease claims boss' (*Sun*, 8 February 1985); 'Hotel bans gay chef who took AIDS test' (*Sun*, 14 February 1985). Cases were also reported, but rarely substantiated according to union officials, of workers refusing to carry out emergency procedures — 'Scared firemen ban the kiss of life' (*Daily Mirror*, 19 February 1985); 'AIDS: Now ambulancemen ban kiss of life' (*Daily Mirror*, 19 February 1985). Even the church was seen as lending its authority to claims of high infectivity via saliva when the *Daily Telegraph* (9 April 1985) ran the headline 'Vicar bows to AIDS fears over chalice'.

Parallel headlines not only suggested that AIDS was highly infectious but also contagious — '"Burn all your clothes" shock at AIDS hospital' (*Sunday Mirror*, 10 February 1985); 'Village fears over AIDS clinic' (*News of the World*, 10 February 1985). Events were also reported which showed that the medical profession itself was not immune to such anxieties —

'Doctor refuses to touch AIDS victim's body' (*Daily Mail*, 16 January 1985); 'Pathologist refused to handle AIDS man's body' (*The Times*, 16 January 1985).

Alongside these accounts were more serious efforts by the press to put across 'the facts' about AIDS in informational features, usually in question and answer, or fact and fiction, format. With varying degrees of success, these features have tried to make it clear that though HIV has been isolated from saliva under laboratory conditions, there is no evidence that it is transmitted this way in everyday life. The *Daily Mail* (17 January 1985) for example in an article headed 'Myths that scare even the doctors' asked, 'Can it spread by kissing or coughing?' to which the reply was given, 'Evidence suggests that, although the virus may be present in saliva, it is not usually infectious when it is'. And readers of *The Times* (21 February 1985) were told under the headline 'What experts know about AIDS' that 'Whilst it is true that the virus has been found in saliva, there is no evidence that the disease can be transmitted from plates or cups, sharing meals or casual contact'. Other newspapers have been less convincing in their treatment of these issues. The *Daily Express* (17 January 1985) for example responded in answer to the question 'Can you catch it by kissing an AIDS victim or by drinking from the same cup?', 'The answer appears to be "No". But small amounts have been identified in saliva, and it is not yet known what virus levels are needed to pass on the disease'.

In February 1985, in an attempt to calm public anxiety about the ease with which HIV infection might be spread, the Chief Medical Officer for England was quoted in the *Daily Telegraph* (7 February 1985) as saying, 'You cannot get it from sitting in the same room as or sharing a meal with, a person with AIDS, since it is not transmitted through the air by coughing or sneezing ... It is nonsense to say, as has been suggested, that homosexuals should not eat in restaurants for fear of passing on the disease ... Whilst it is true that the virus has been found in saliva, there is no evidence that the disease has been transmitted from plates or cups'. The same month also saw the Health Education Council publishing its second booklet 'Some facts about AIDS' in which it was stated, 'There is absolutely no reason to think that AIDS can be spread through the air or by touch'.

The impression that these official health education messages conveyed was, however, largely eclipsed by concurrent reports of avoidance behaviour by the public and professionals alike in the popular press. At the best of times it may be difficult for a lay audience to understand complex medical distinctions between infection and contagion, and between *in vitro* and *in vivo* evidence. But the acute contradiction between the more circumspect health education messages on the one hand, and newspaper accounts of the elaborate precautionary measures apparently being taken on the other, made it difficult for many people to assess their own risk of infection in a balanced and responsible way. The idea that the virus is not transmitted in saliva, and that touching carries no risk fails to square easily with potent images of communion chalices being abandoned, clothing being burned and bodies being left unburied. Continued reference to terms such as 'leper' and 'plague' in newspaper reporting of AIDS also reinforced the popular perception that AIDS was in fact a highly contagious disease.

It should, therefore, come as little surprise to learn that when the first official public information campaign about AIDS was finally launched in spring 1986, it made less impact than might have been hoped for. According to a Gallup Poll (*New Society*, 1986) conducted in February and March of that year before the campaign began, 20 per cent of the public still thought they could catch AIDS by being sneezed at, 19 per cent still thought that toilet seats posed a risk and 25 per cent were worried about sharing the same glass with another person. By July and August of the same year after the first stage of the campaign, these proportions had improved only marginally to 16 per cent, 17 per cent and 22 per cent respectively.

Media Representations, Perceptions of Risk and Health Education

At the beginning of this chapter, it was suggested that how people assess their own personal level of risk within the context of a disease such as AIDS depends on who and how many people are perceived to be affected, what the causes of the disease are understood to be, and how the disease is believed to be transmitted. Risk assessment in relation to disease prevention as in any other context involves the dual process of estimating the probabilities of various outcomes and evaluating their consequences (Janis and Mann, 1977). In relation to AIDS, this requires thinking intelligently about low probability events with serious consequences. This is no easy task for those well practised in health-related decision-making, let alone for ordinary women and men, and an essential pre-requisite for this kind of thought is good information.

As we have seen, in the case of AIDS this is clearly problematic in at least two related ways. First, whilst knowledge of the disease is accumulating rapidly, and is constantly being revised as more clinical, social and epidemiological information becomes available, many aspects of the etiology of AIDS are still unclear. As Coxon's chapter elsewhere in this book makes clear, the answers to questions about how far and how fast HIV infection will spread beyond currently identified 'high risk' groups, for example, are as yet based largely on informed guesswork. Further biases can also be built into our understanding of AIDS by the manner in which particular areas of study are selected, by the ways in which observations are made, by the way in which data is subsequently analyzed and by how the research findings are reported.

Second, even given these imperfections in the information we have, there is still ample opportunity for distortion to take place during its dissemination. Except in a few cases, members of the public are unlikely to have access to primary source data about AIDS — they must rely instead on second and third hand reports for their information. The national press therefore has a particularly powerful role to play in mediating between available scientific evidence on the one hand and public perceptions of AIDS on the other. Within this context, we have already seen how misunderstandings have been generated via the selective attention this section of the media has given to particular sorts of material as the basis for its news stories and features; via the ways in which scientific evidence has been interpreted and presented; and via the use of emphasis and the playing up of certain 'angles' in the reporting of AIDS stories.

These misunderstandings would not be so serious if they did not have profound consequences for the extent to which individuals may perceive themselves (and others) to be at risk of HIV infection and/or AIDS, and for the extent to which they have confused scientific analysis with moral prescription.

With respect to perceptions of risk, it is possible to tentatively identify some of the consequences that have followed media reports of AIDS such as those described. In order to do this, I will use an analytic framework put forward by Tversky and Kahnemann (1974) to identify some of the popular misunderstandings that national press reporting of AIDS may have helped establish. In situations where there exists doubt and uncertainty, people use a variety of mental techniques or 'short cuts' to handle the information they are presented with. These heuristics generally serve us well in 'making sense' of complex and contradictory information, but in some circumstances they can lead to bias and error in our perceptions of the world.

According to Tversky and Kahnemann, one heuristic which is particularly relevant to the discussion of AIDS is that of *availability*. This prompts us to assign a higher probability of occurrence to those events which are easier to imagine or recall than to those which are not. How easily we can imagine or recall an event depends on how recently the information was acquired (Tversky and Kahnemann call this the 'recency effect') and what sort of impact it had on us (they call this the 'emotional saliency' effect). Generally speaking, *availability* is an effective guide to probability assessment since likely occurrences are easier to imagine than unlikely ones. However, where the apparent frequency of a particular event is greater than its actual frequency, and where the emotional import of an event is exagerrated, reliance on this heuristic may lead us to overestimate the probability of certain events occurring.

Thus the regular bombardment of public consciousness with highly emotive images would arguably form a stronger input into public perceptions of risk than would a more sporadic, measured and low key form of health educational intervention. Further, the singling out of certain events for attention disproportionate to their relative incidence (the 'accidental' transmission of HIV via blood or blood products, for example), and their investment with higher emotional significance, can result in the chances of HIV transmission by this means being greatly overestimated by the public.

A second cognitive bias discussed by Tversky and Kahnemann is the *representative* bias. This stems from lack of background information about a particular issue compared with foreground information. By the term background information is meant information about the distribution of relative characteristics in a particular population, and by the term foreground information is meant information about a particular case. Typically background information comes in the form of base rates, neglect of which prompts generalizations from specific instances to all cases. This temptation to make inferences from small unrepresentative numbers can be found in media reports estimating the prevalence of HIV infection in the gay population by extrapolating from highly select sub-groups of this population (London STD clinic attenders, for example). At its most extreme, this bias can lead to an almost syllogistic mode of reasoning — that AIDS predominantly strikes gay men, therefore all gay men are stricken with AIDS. Both in terms of press comment and public reaction, AIDS and gay sexuality have at times seemed to be coterminous and interchangeable, as the ostracization of gay men at places of work and recreation demonstrates (these points are discussed at greater length in Robertson's chapter in this book).

Tversky and Kahnemann's third heuristic, the *anchoring* mechanism, has possibly the most pessimistic implications for realistic assessments of risk within the context of HIV infection and AIDS. According to this, people attach disproportionate importance to their initial assessments of risk. This hampers their ability to make revisions in this in the light of new information. In terms of national press reporting, we can find evidence of this bias in the apparent reluctance of feature writers and editors over the period 1983 to 1985 to reformulate their theories about the causation of AIDS, as well as in their resistance to evidence critical of the (quite unwarranted) notion that AIDS was an exclusively gay disease. At the level of public perception, this is a bias which also has particularly gloomy implications for health education. If we accept that an anchoring mechanism is likely to operate within popular assessments of risk, then the long gap between the first onslaught of media publicity about AIDS (with its emphasis on the 'gayness' of the disease) and later more wide ranging health education initiatives, will have limited the impact and effectiveness of these latter messages and their ability to change attitudes and judgments.

Conclusions

In this chapter efforts have been made to identify some of the systematic biases that can be found in British national newspaper reporting of AIDS between 1983 and 1985. I have also tried to explore some of the possible consequences of these for popular perceptions of risk as well as for the effectiveness (or otherwise) of more recent health education initiatives. From the evidence presented, there would seem to be good reason to believe that the effectiveness of health education relating to AIDS may be hampered in the immediate future by misunderstandings created and reinforced by national newspaper coverage of AIDS. By and large, this has been far from accurate in its identification of the causes of AIDS, the scale of the epidemic, the groups most affected by it and the means by which the disease is transmitted.

In the light of this, we should remain vigilant in our appraisal of the content of newspaper articles relating to AIDS. Health educators in particular have an important role to play in correcting misleading reporting and emphases as well as in providing newspapers with press release information relating to new interventions and initiatives.

Notes

1 See for example PIOT, P., TAELMAN, H., MANLANGU, K. B. *et al.* (1984) 'Acquired immunodeficiency syndrome in a heterosexual population in Zaire'.

Lancet, ii, pp 65–9; DE COCK, K.M. (1984) 'AIDS: An old disease from Africa', *British Medical Journal*, ii, pp 306–8.
2 Personal communication with Dr Anthony Pinching, St Mary's Hospital, London.

References

ALTER, H. J., EICHBERG, J. W., MASUR, H. *et al* (1984) 'Transmission of HTLV-II infection from human plasma to chimpanzees: An animal model for AIDS', *Science*, 11 November, pp 549–52.

ALTMAN, D. (1986) *AIDS and the New Puritanism*, London, Auto Press.

CLUMECK, N. *et al* (1983) 'Acquired Immune Deficiency Syndrome in Black Africans', *Lancet*, i, p 642.

FELSTEIN, I. (1974) *Sexual Pollution: The Rise and Fall of Venereal Diseases*, London, David and Charles.

GOEDERT, J. J., NEULAND, C. Y., WALLERN, W. C. *et al* (1982) 'Amyl nitrite may alter T-lymphocytes in homosexual men', *Lancet*, i, pp 412–6.

GROOPMAN, J. E., SALAHUDDIN, S. Z., SARNGADHARAN, M. G. *et al* (1984) 'HTLV-III in saliva of people with AIDS related complex and healthy homosexual men at risk for AIDS', *Science*, 226, 4673, pp 447–9.

GYORKEY, F., SINKOVICS, J. G., GYORKEY, P. *et al* (1982) 'Tuboreticular structures in Kaposi's sarcoma', *Lancet*, ii, p 984.

HSIA, S., SHOCKLEY, R. K., LUTCHER, C. L. *et al* (1984) 'Unregulated production of a virus and/or sperm specific anti-idiotypic antibodies as a cause of AIDS', *Lancet*, ii, pp 212–4.

JANIS, I. and MANN, L. (1977) *Decision Making: A Psychological Analysis of Conflict, Choice and Commitment*, New York, Free Press.

JORGENSON, K. A. (1982) 'Amyl nitrite and Kaposi's sarcoma in homosexual men', *New England Journal of Medicine*, 307. pp 893–4.

LACEY, C. J. N. and WAUGH, M. A. (1983) 'Cellular immunity in male homosexuals', *Lancet*, ii, p 464.

MCEVOY, M. and TILLETT, H. (1985) 'AIDS for all by the year 2000?', *British Medical Journal*, 290, i, p 463.

MARMOR, M., LAUBENSTEIN, L., WILLIAM, D. C. *et al* (1982) 'Risk factors for Kaposi's sarcoma in homosexual men', *Lancet*, i, p 1083–7.

MORTIMER, P. P., JESSON, W. J., VANDERWELDE, E. M. *et al* (1985) 'Prevalence of antibody to Human T lymphotropic virus type III by risk group and area, United Kingdom 1978–84', *British Medical Journal*, 290, i, pp 1176–80.

New Scientist (1983) 'AIDS: the homosexual connection', 1 December.

New Society (1986) 'Gallup Poll findings on AIDS', 29 August, p 5.

OSWALD, G. A., THEODOSSI, A., GAZZARD, B. G. *et al* (1982) 'Attempted immune stimulation in the "gay compromise syndrome"', *British Medical Journal*, ii, p 1082.

PINCHING, A. J., JEFFRIES, D. J., DONAGHY, M. *et al* (1983) 'Studies of cellular immunity in male homosexuals in London', *Lancet*, ii, pp 126–30.

ROSE, D. B. and KEYSTONE, J. S. (1983) 'AIDS in a Canadian woman who helped prostitutes in Port-au-Prince', *Lancet*, ii, pp 680–1.

SMITH, C. L., BUCKLEY, P. M., HELLIWELL, T. R. *et al* (1983) 'AIDS in a woman in England', *Lancet*, ii, p 846.

TVERSKY, A. and KAHNEMANN, D. (1974) 'Judgment under uncertainty', *Science*, 185, pp 1124–31.

WATERSON, A. P. (1983) 'Acquired Immune Deficiency Syndrome', *British Medical Journal*, i, pp 743–6.

6
Young People's Health Beliefs and AIDS

Ian Warwick, Peter Aggleton and Hilary Homans

Explanations of health, illness and disease are diverse. Some of these define health in negative terms as either the absence of disease or the absence of illness, while others take a more positive expansionist position by suggesting that health may be more appropriately defined as the presence of certain qualities. Perhaps the best known of definition of this latter kind is that put forward by the World Health Organization in 1946. This suggested that 'health is a state of complete physical, mental and social well-being' (WHO, 1946).

Until recently, the professional understandings of health that doctors and other health professionals share have conceptualized health as the absence of disease. According to mainstream professional explanations, people become sick largely as a result of their bodies having been 'invaded' by external agents such as bacteria, viruses and protozoa. Biomedical understandings such as these stress the need for sophisticated clinical tests to determine the effects of pathological microorganisms. They also emphasize the value of research into chemotherapeutic 'cures' for disease.

Recent developments in community health, as well as in alternative and complementary medicine, have questioned the usefulness of explanations which privilege the biological determinants and correlates of health and well-being above those which are social and psychological in their nature. McIntyre's (1986) work, for example, suggests that rarely is there a clear cut relationship between the physical indices of disease and the subjective experience of illness and distress. People can, for example, feel 'well' even when a physical examination would show them to be severely 'diseased'. Similarly, it is quite possible for a person to 'feel ill' in the absence of identifiable cell pathology.

In the light of this, social researchers as well as doctors (Helman,

1978) have increasingly turned their attention to exploring the ways in which health and illness are subjectively experienced. Co-existing with professional explanations and definitions are popular or lay beliefs about health. These are generally *syncretic* in their origins, being derived from a variety of disparate sources (Fitzpatrick, 1984). At least five different kinds of lay beliefs about health and illness have been identified. These 'explain' (i) the etiology of sickness; (ii) the factors associated with the onset of symptoms; (iii) the pathophysiology that is assumed to be taking place; (iv) the course that the sickness is likely to take; and (v) the most appropriate kind of treatment (Kleinman, 1976). It is important to recognize, however, that lay beliefs about health and illness do not arise from either ignorance or the wilful misinterpretation of mainstream medical knowledge. They are actively constructed in an effort to 'make sense' of the frequently confusing and contradictory experiences that people have. Indeed, there is often a degree of overlap between lay and professional explanations, with health professionals themselves subscribing to both lay and professional beliefs (Helman, 1978), and lay beliefs being influenced by those advances in medical knowledge which are more popularly known about.

The External Relations of Lay Beliefs about Health and Illness

We have already argued that lay beliefs about health and illness help people 'make sense' of the various events that befall them. It is important to recognize that lay health beliefs relate not only to the personal biography of the individual who adheres to them, but to more enduring cultural and social structures. There is a growing literature, for example, which identifies racial, class and gender differences in the ways in which people conceptualize and understand health and illness (Seabrook, 1973; McKeown, 1979; Graham, 1984; d'Houtard and Field, 1984; Homans, 1985; Donovan, 1986; Hart, 1985).

Lay health beliefs are therefore constituted through complex cultural processes involving active interplay between dominant and dominated systems of meaning. In this respect, it should come as little surprise to find that people's lay beliefs about health relate closely to the social strategies that they conventionally use to negotiate contradictions associated with their social position. A recent study by Pill and Scott (1982) clearly demonstrates this. In their interviews with women with childcare responsibilities, Pill and Scott were concerned to explore why their respondents were apparently 'resisting' efforts being made at the time by the Department of Health and Social Security to encourage them to accept greater personal responsibility for their own health. Only a minority of the women interviewed shared a commitment to this perspective. The majority displayed considerable antipathy to the suggestion that they should take the same responsibility for their own health as they did for that of their children, arguing that their role as 'mothers' necessitated that they provide differentially for themselves and for their children. Pill and Scott interpret their findings in terms of a tension between conformity towards notions of 'motherhood' and notions of 'personal responsibility'.

Similarly, Graham (1984) has argued that it is the woman's health which suffers most in her attempts to cope with the pressures of home and family. Tranquilizers and smoking are both used to lessen stress and to enable mothers to remain calm and 'cope' with demanding situations. Jacobson (1981) has also argued that smoking may provide a way in which women can create a space and time for themselves away from family constraints.

The Internal Dynamics of Lay Beliefs about Health and Illness

A considerable amount of effort has been invested in identifying the kinds of lay explanation that are recurrently used to explain health and sickness. Research of this type has identified the internal structure of a variety of modes of analysis widely employed in 'making sense' of health-related conditions. Herzlich (1973), for example, in her study of middle class Parisians has identified three different ways in which health is popularly understood. First there is a notion of health as a *state of being* in which there was a clear absence of disease. This understanding shares an affinity with contemporary biomedical definitions of health. Then there is an understanding of health as a *quality to be had* — be this robustness, strength or resistance to infection. Finally, she identifies a lay understanding of health as a *state of doing*.

With respect to lay understandings of illness, Herzlich has identified three different kinds of explanation. She suggests that illness can be popularly understood as *destructive* (in the sense that it isolates individuals and destroys their existing social relationships), as *liberatory* (in the sense that it can provide opportunities for solitude and contemplation that might otherwise be denied) and as an *occupation* (in the sense that those concerned might pursue appropriate 'careers' involving recourse to professional advice and active involvement in achieving the desired goal of recovery).

Other studies have identified a difference between lay theories of illness causation which emphasize internal or *endogenous* factors and those which emphasize external *exogenous* ones (Herzlich and Pierret, 1986). Further lay explanations emphasize *personal responsibility*, or more usually *personal irresponsibility*, as a factor leading to the onset of illness (Illsley *et al*, 1977; Helman, 1978; Zola, 1966). *Supernatural intervention* too is sometimes invoked within lay theories about sickness. The origins of many modern retributionist analysis of illness causation can be traced back to the causes of ill-health identified in early Christian dogma (Unschuld, 1986).

Lay Beliefs about Health and AIDS

There are a number of reasons why lay health beliefs should be of importance to social and health researchers within the context of HIV infection and AIDS. First, lay beliefs about health and illness are likely to act as powerful mediators of official health education messages which rely on professional and biomedical explanations to inform people about the causes of HIV infection and/or AIDS. Second, popular understandings of health may have a significant role to play in influencing people's perceptions of the 'risks' associated with particular social situations and particular social and sexual acts. Third, they may affect the ways in which changes in health status — be these AIDS-related or otherwise — are experienced.

Whilst a number of studies have now been published which identify people's acquaintance (or non-acquaintance) with mainstream professional understandings of AIDS (Mills *et al*, 1987; Searle, 1987), there are relatively few studies which have investigated people's lay beliefs about HIV infection and AIDS. Rarer still are investigations of the beliefs that young people in particular hold about AIDS.

In one of the earliest papers of its type, Bolognone and Johnson (1986) begin an exploration of the relationship between professional explanatory models of AIDS and the lay beliefs they elicited during interviews with lesbians and gay men as well as with members of what they call the 'non-gay sector'. They discovered that the lay beliefs of lesbians and gay men showed greater congruence with mainstream professional explanations than did those of non-gay women and men. Personal communication, particularly with physicians, seemed to be a particularly potent source of information affecting the lay beliefs that these respondents had about AIDS.

A recent study by DiClemente *et al* (1986) of young people's attitudes and beliefs about AIDS conducted in the San Francisco area highlights the uneven levels of knowledge about HIV infection and AIDS that can be found among young people. Although 92 per cent of those interviewed agreed that 'sexual intercourse was one mode of contracting AIDS' (sic), there was still considerable confusion about the ways in which the risk of infection could be minimized. For example, small but significant numbers of young people continue to believe that AIDS (sic) can be transmitted by touching, kissing or being near an infected person. The authors of this chapter conclude somewhat pessimistically that residence close to what they refer to as a 'high density AIDS epicenter' is no guarantee of high levels of awareness about the causes of AIDS.

In their study of lay beliefs about AIDS conducted in Britain, Clift and Stears (1987) interviewed a range of college students before and after the major public information campaign launched by the Department of Health at the end of 1986. They were unable to identify significant differences between the lay beliefs of young women and young men in their sample, but found that worry about contracting AIDS (sic) via casual contact and moral perceptions of AIDS were more prevalent among religious, right-wing, exclusively heterosexual students than amongst others.

It is important to recognize, however, that the majority of studies identifying people's lay beliefs about AIDS have used pre-structured approaches to data collection. Within this paradigm, respondents are most usually asked to indicate their agreement or disagreement with 'ready made' statements about HIV infection and/or AIDS. Whilst it can be plausibly argued that the statements to be found in AIDS awareness questionnaires do indeed bear a relation to the kinds of lay beliefs about AIDS that people share, research of this kind needs to be complemented by more interpretative studies which set out to explore the complexity and contradictoriness of health knowledge about AIDS. In this chapter, therefore, and by way of contrast with much of the published research, we will report on preliminary findings from an in-depth study of young people's lay beliefs about HIV infection and AIDS. The data we will present has been collected as part of a research project which has used qualitative methodology to explore young people's perceptions of AIDS.

The Young People's Health Knowledge and AIDS Project

In September 1986, we began an in-depth study of lay beliefs about HIV infection and AIDS as a prelude to a more wide ranging survey of the ways in which AIDS and HIV infection are commonly understood. In connection with this in-depth work we have interviewed forty-three young people aged between 16 and 21 participating in local authority youth provision and youth training schemes (YTS) in selected urban areas in northern and south-west England. Most of the youth clubs, drop in centres and other youth facilities in which we have carried out fieldwork have been community based — drawing their membership from young people living in their immediate vicinity. A few, however, have been specifically designated by the local authority funding their activities as concerned with the needs of young lesbians and young gay men. In this chapter, we will not report on our findings from lesbian and gay youth groups but will restrict our attention to the health beliefs of young people attending community based youth groups and YTS programmes.

We negotiated access to youth and community provision through area youth officers who were sent details of the project as well as our research intentions. This information was subsequently distributed to youth workers in the field who were asked whether they would be interested in participating in the project. In the light of the interest shown, two youth groups were initially approached and a meeting arranged between the youth worker responsible for their activities and a member of the project team (Ian Warwick). During these initial consultations it became clear that youth workers were concerned that those interviewed should subsequently benefit from their involvement in the project, and it was agreed that project findings would be disseminated back to the young people who had participated in the enquiry via workshops, newsletters, group and individual discussions. Access to young people participating in YTS provision on the other hand was gained via links between the project and local voluntary sector organizations providing AIDS-related education support and counselling.

In view of the exploratory nature of the study and our desire to explore in depth young people's beliefs about AIDS, data was collected via tape recorded semi-structured interviews. Because of our concern to examine popular perceptions of HIV infection and its consequences within the context of lay beliefs about health and illness in general, a series of open-ended questions were constructed to enquire into young people's beliefs about a wide range of health related issues including the common cold, spots, cancer, sexually transmitted diseases and so on. Additionally, a series of question was identified which addressed specific beliefs about HIV infection and/or AIDS. In order to enhance the naturalism of the present enquiry, these questions were introduced in a variety of ways depending upon the expectations of the young people concerned. On some occasions, and in keeping with the ethos of the activities within the youth facility concerned, the questions were presented on cards to be chosen and responded to by each member of the group in turn. On other occasions, when it would have been unduly artificial to collect data in this way, the questions were introduced within the context of general discussions about health and illness.

Group-based interviews were carried out wherever possible lasting approximately an hour. Care was taken to ensure that more time than this was available should it be required since it was discovered early in the fieldwork that many of the young people interviewed welcomed the chance to talk about their more general fears and anxieties with respect to HIV infection and AIDS. The twenty-three young people whose views are reported in this paper varied in age from 16 to 21, there being an equal mix of women and men.

In our interviews with young people about AIDS we were concerned to explore a variety of interrelated issues. First we were interested in identifying how young people *conceptualized* HIV infection and AIDS. Second, we were interested in identifying what young people perceived as the *immediate 'causes' of AIDS*. Were these perceived as being viral in nature? Or were they perceived as the consequences of certain acts (sexual or otherwise) or of contact with specific categories of person? Third, we were concerned to identify what young people felt were the *ultimate origins* of AIDS above and beyond its immediate 'causes'.[1] Finally, we were interested in identifying resonances and tensions between young people's understandings of AIDS and their understandings of other forms of sickness.

Young People's Conceptualization of HIV Infection and AIDS

'The Virus' and 'the AIDS'

In order to begin our exploration of young people's beliefs about AIDS, we asked them what they thought AIDS was. Most of those we talked to seemed confident of one thing. AIDS is above all damaging and destructive — a 'killer disease' as many put it.

IW:	What is AIDS?
Steve:	Death.
Owen:	A killer disease isn't it? It can't be cured, so it's a killer.
Gill:	What is AIDS? The only thing I can say is that AIDS is a killer.

Some (but not all) of the young people we interviewed were able to identify a viral etiology for the syndrome. In this respect, it is interesting to note that their responses mirrored those of the adult respondents interviewed in Vass's (1986) study of beliefs about AIDS.

Jas: By all accounts there's a certain monkey in Africa that actually carries the virus ...

IW: OK, so there's a virus?.

Jas: Yeah, there's actually a virus.

The majority of those we have interviewed seem quite unable to distinguish between having HIV infection and developing AIDS. Indeed, even amongst those who talked separately of a virus (the 'AIDS virus' as it was usually called) and AIDS there was considerable confusion as the following makes clear.

IW: ... like I was saying, you can't catch the virus from cups.

Steve: But can you get *the actual AIDS* from cups?

IW: No, because to get AIDS you ...

Steve: ... I know, you need the virus, but say somebody had the virus and they gradually got on to AIDS and they had a cup and you drank out of it afterwards, then you couldn't catch the virus?

IW: No, the, I don't quite know what you're saying.

Steve: All right, somebody has the virus right? And it gradually gets on to AIDS right? They drink out of a cup and then you drink out of it after. Like you're sort of sharing a cup right? 'Do you want a drink' yeah? Can't you catch the virus?

IW: No.

Steve: So you can't catch nothing? You can't catch the virus and you can't catch AIDS?

Steve, like other young people we talked to, drew a distinction between getting 'the virus' and getting something else which he calls 'the actual AIDS'. Whilst by the end of this interview he seemed relatively confident that 'the virus' could not be transmitted via shared cups and cutlery, we were left with the feeling (and this was after strenuous efforts had been made to convince him otherwise) that he still had doubts about whether something else — 'the actual AIDS' — might not be transmitted this way.[2] Given the consistent failure to distinguish between HIV infection and AIDS in media reporting of AIDS, it is hardly surprising that views like these continue to be expressed. The fact that they are, however, raises important questions about the effectiveness of recent public information campaigns which have attempted to alleviate unreasonable levels of anxiety.

Attacking, Fighting and Destroying

Militaristic imagery recurred frequently in young people's descriptions of HIV infection and AIDS. Our respondents often suggested that AIDS damages the 'defences' of the body, so leaving a person unable to resist further 'attack'. Imagery involving notions of 'fighting', 'killing', 'defending' and 'destroying' was used a great deal in talking about AIDS. This conceptualization of the body-as-battleground is of course a peculiarly modern way of expressing concern about germs and the effects they may have, and this is one which has become the dominant mode of analysis within mainstream medical explanation (Sontag, 1979; Patton, 1985).

Sue: Well, you don't actually die from AIDS anyway 'cos what it is ... it's a virus that *breaks down* your *resistance*.

IW: So you die from other things?

Sue: And it *kills* your *resistance*, but you don't actually die from AIDS. You can die from bronchitis or pneumonia or something like that.

In a similar way, Joe argued that,

Joe: AIDS *destroys* your immune system ... you die of something else entirely.

and Terri claimed,

Terri: (AIDS) *kills off* one lot of cells and leaves the other cells *defenceless* and therefore your body doesn't just die from AIDS, it's a disease that puts you at risk from anything else, cuts down your chance of survival from it and you can die from more or less anything else. (emphasis added)

Having AIDS

During the course of our interviews we were also concerned to ask young people what they would do if they were to be diagnosed with either HIV infection or AIDS. A common response to this question emphasized their concern not to 'pass' either of these states of being on to other people.

Steve: What would I do if I had AIDS? Stop sleeping about. There's not a lot you can do once you've got it. Don't give it to anyone else at all.

Some young people considered taking more drastic steps than this. Although respondents sometimes joked about whether they would 'top themselves', there were also serious discussions about whether or not suicide might be preferable to living with HIV infection or AIDS.

IW: What would you do if you had the virus?
Karen: Commit suicide.
IW: Would you?
Karen: (laughing) Yeah.
IW: Why's that?
Karen: Because I, you know, I wouldn't want to pass it on to anybody else and I, I just wouldn't want to be a burden to anybody. I wouldn't want to go through all that pain. So really I'd just commit suicide. I'd just take an overdose. It's not fair on your family. You don't want to be a burden on anyone. I wouldn't want to pass it on to nobody else. Anyway, it's embarrassing.

The disruption to existing social relationships, the potential 'embarrassment' of being diagnosed with either HIV infection and/or AIDS, as well as the social isolation that might then ensue, were all important factors to be taken into account in deciding whether or not to inform others.

Sue: I wouldn't tell no one. I wouldn't tell no one, because you know some people they're childish. They'll say 'Get away from me' You know what I mean?
Earl: Depends ... It really is wrong not to let other people know. But again, if you let people know, they see, to treat you as an outcast, don't want to know you, you could get the sack. Er, it's like, you see on the telly people who said ... they've been telling people who're still working, if you've got AIDS not to tell your employers 'cos it will ...
Lee: ... ruin you life ...
Earl: ... will probably affect your job. But they're trying to put it through a tribunal or something where they can't do nothing about it.
Lee: If you had a wife and kids and you had AIDS and your boss or employer found out, and he was going to sack you, and your wife was going to leave you, you'd have lost everything.

Young people's beliefs about how they might be treated by others were they to be diagnosed as 'having AIDS' contrasted dramatically with the ways in which they said they would treat someone they knew if they developed the syndrome.

Steve: Well, I'd try and support him the best I could. I'd help the best way I could. It's all you can do really. Give him moral support.

Joe: Well, it's easy for me to say that I'd try and help him but ... er ... I'm not sure if I'd feel like many other people ... er ... who've known someone who's had AIDS and (who) treat them like outcasts. You can't really say (though) until you've actually known someone. But if ... I think I'd try and help them as much as I could like.

Jill: How would you feel if someone you knew had the virus and what would you do? Well, I wouldn't ... some people when they find out they leave their friends, but I wouldn't do that. I'd stick by them and help them through it I suppose. It's all you can do.

So far we have discussed some of the ways in which the young people we interviewed 'made sense' of AIDS as a medical, social and cultural phenomenon. We will now turn our attention to some of the lay explanations about the cause of AIDS that young people operate with. Our fieldwork has suggested that in this respect it is useful to distinguish between those systems of belief which address the factors that might explain why a particular individual may (or may not) acquire HIV infection and/or AIDS (we will call these lay theories of immediate causation) and those which address more general questions about the ultimate origins of AIDS as a disease (we will call these lay theories of ultimate causation).

Lay Theories of Immediate Causation

When we asked young people what factors might more immediately lead to a person developing AIDS, a number of kinds of explanation were offered. Some of these emphasized *exogenous* variables, whereas others emphasized more *endogenous* factors.

Exogenous theories of disease causation assign primacy to factors which are external to the individual. These can include climate, bad air and germs. Within respect to lay beliefs of immediate causation, we found that the young people we interviewed used two types of exogenous explanation. The first, which we have already mentioned, stressed that in reality either 'AIDS' or 'the virus' is highly contagious. It can therefore be passed on by drinking out of the same glass as someone else or by sharing a cigarette provided that someone with 'the virus' or with 'AIDS' has just used that object. Some of our interviewees went so far as to suggest that touch alone might be sufficient to ensure transmission.

Mary: Oh sure you can get it from touching, being in the same place as someone else, brushing up against them like. That's why it's so frightening really.

For some young people this first kind of exogenous explanation links closely to a second set of lay theories of immediate causation. These suggest that 'AIDS' or 'the virus' lies in wait, lurking unseen and ready to infect.

Steve: There's a lot of it around, this AIDS. It's everywhere. You get it from the environment you live in, (from) the people you mix with and what have you.

Miasmatic beliefs like these seem to be closely related both to the apparent invisibility both of the virus itself, and of people who have HIV infection and/or AIDS. The idea that there may be 'carriers' of the disease (a notion heavily reinforced by recent media reporting of AIDS) emphasizes for some young people the difficulty of telling who may or may not have been infected, and when and where contact with the virus is most likely to take place.

Concurrent with beliefs such as these were others which suggested that personal qualities inherent in the individual might make them particularly susceptible to infection. In discussing these *endogenous* theories, our data suggests that it is important to distinguish between those explanations which individuals use to 'make sense' of the events that befall others and those which they use to 'make sense' of events affecting their own lives.

When it comes to explaining events that happen to others, pervasive systems of belief which distiguish between so-called 'innocent' and 'guilty' 'victims' of the disease are called upon.[3] These distinctions differentiate between those whose behaviour 'makes it reasonable' that they should have developed AIDS and those who have developed the syndrome 'through no fault of their own'. Gay men, prostitutes, the 'promiscuous', bisexuals and injecting drug users are usually incorporated within the first of these categories, whereas haemophiliacs, children, the married partners of those who engage in extra-marital relationships and the recipients of blood transfusions are generally given prominence within the second (Altman, 1986; Watney, 1987; Wellings, 1987).

Amongst the young people we have talked to, these distinctions are used quite unproblematically. Indeed, when we asked our respondents to consider what they would do if one of their friends developed AIDS, some suggested that the first thing on their agenda would be to determine which of the categories 'innocent' or 'guilty' best described the situation.

Colin: Well, if I found out that one of my friends had the virus then it's question time ... How did he catch it, who was he with and all that, you know? It's serious, it's question time. How long have you had it? All that, you know what I mean?

IW: Would it matter how he got it?

Colin: It depends how he got it. You know, if he just got it from straight sex, there ain't nothing wrong with that. (But) if he got it in a different way, like he was holding on to another man, well, he's got his conscience to think about. I mean, come off it man, he's bound to get rushed, he's bound to get laughed at, dubbed and all that crap. You know what I mean?

This line of analysis was extended further in another interview.

Jo: Well, most of them are innocent but, you know, they're telling you that it's a bad thing to have sex and some people aren't listeing to it. If you're going to sleep around then ...

Mary: ... You know you're going to get it in the end

Curiously, when young people were asked to reflect on events that might affect their own lives (rather than those of others) a switch of logic took place with the emphasis being placed far more on luck or chance than on *personal responsibility*.

Phil: You can get AIDS sleeping around with women, with men, like you said — blood transfusions. You might catch it from being dirty. I never know. If you've got AIDS, you've got AIDS. That's life.

Jas: Who gets the virus? I dunno. It's just the unlucky person innit?

IW: Right, so it's luck?

Jas: Bad luck, I think!

— laughter —

Jas: Bad luck whoever gets it. I can't think who gets it 'cos anybody can get it I suppose.

IW: Can you stop yourself from getting it?

Jas: I dunno. 'Cos you can get it from different ways innit? 'Cos I heard that you can get it from drinking out of that person's cup and if you don't know that person's got the virus and you drink out of the cup then you've got it haven't you?

This disjunction between the logic used to explain why certain categories of others (normally the supposedly 'guilty' victims identified earlier) might develop AIDS and that used to explain all other cases was shown particularly clearly in a claim made by Tim.

Tim: Some people ... You can make yourself more at risk if you're a homosexual or a junkie, or both at the same time. You're at highest risk then and you could expect to get it. But if you're heterosexual and you're not a junkie, if you catch it (then) you're really unlucky.

This statement, however, raises yet further questions about the ways in which an essentially *serendipitous* logic is used to 'make sense' of AIDS. It would seem from the claim that Tim makes that 'luck' and 'chance' operate only to explain heterosexual transmission. Heterosexuals can not logically 'expect to get it', so when they do, it must be because of 'chance' or 'bad luck', and not through any 'fault' or their own. This belief may have important implications for some young people's perceptions of risk, since it suggests that perceptions of risk (in the case of men at least) may be mediated by whether or not they self-identify as heterosexual or gay. Since there is now considerable evidence to suggest that many men who participate in homosexual acts do not consider themselves to be anything other than heterosexual (Reiss, 1961; Humphreys, 1970; Weinberg, 1983), our findings raise important questions about the relationship between sexual identity and risk perception.

Lay Theories of Ultimate Causation

In our discussions with young people we were concerned to move beyond the immediate factors that they felt were involved in the causation of AIDS to identify lay beliefs about what were perceived as the ultimate origins of the syndrome. Three rather different kinds of explanation seemed evident here. Two of these were broadly exogenous in nature. The first emphasized *environmental disturbance*, the second *supernatural intervention*. A third lay theory of this type suggested that the ultimate origins of AIDS may be found as an *essence* within us all.

Lay analyses of the former type suggested that AIDS may have originated as a result of attempts to 'meddle with the environment'. The testing of too many atomic weapons, the introduction of atomic power as well as the pollution of the environment by chemical wastes were all seen as having created an ecological instability resulting in AIDS.

Marlene: Well I think there's a lot of truth about this pollution business. All these weapons and things, nuclear power ... it messes up the environment so it's no wonder then that AIDS appears.

In contrast to recent statements by editorial writers within the popular press (*The Times*, 1984), conservative social commentators (Anderson, 1986) and Chief Constables of Police (*The Guardian*, 1986) only two of the young people we talked to suggested that the ultimate origin of AIDS might be supernatural.

Robert: If you really want to know what I think about AIDS, I think it's been sent to us by God. Not to punish us but to warn us not to go too far, but to return to the scriptures, to lead good lives ... that's what I think.

Early in our work, we were somewhat surprised to identify a third, and at the time quite unanticipated, lay theory of ultimate causation. This suggests that AIDS (like cancer so these same respondents told us) may be already present in every person. Like the creatures in the film *Alien*, AIDS lurks opportunistically within us, simply waiting the right moment to make its presence known.

Jill: AIDS? People are born with it. It's in them from the start. It's something you carry without even knowing it ... rather like cancer really. I was watching this film the other day about that, like we've all got it in us right from the start.

The Relationship Between Understandings of AIDS and Understandings of Other Disease

Of particular interest to us has been the extent to which young people's beliefs about AIDS mirror those that have been identified with respect to other diseases. Our descriptions of the ways in which respondents conceptualized AIDS as well as the beliefs they held about the immediate and ultimate causes of the syndrome suggest that there is some degree of match between lay beliefs about AIDS and those to do with other diseases. In our own interviews, for example, we have identified lay theories which emphasize *endogenous* and *exogenous* factors, *personal responsibility* and *supernatural intervention*. We have also confirmed that young people's lay beliefs about HIV infection and AIDS are on occasion influenced by notions of *miasma* and contagion. These findings are clearly resonant with recurrent themes to be found in the growing literature on lay health beliefs in general (Helman, 1978; Herzlich and Pierret, 1986; Unschuld, 1986).

Another way in which young people's beliefs about AIDS paralleled more generally identified lay understandings of illness can be found in the extent to which AIDS is almost universally seen as *destructive*. Such a view contrasted sharply with the ways in which these same young people conceptualized the common cold and sexually transmitted diseases other than HIV infection. The common cold, for example, was usually construed as *liberatory* (since it provided an opportunity for respite from the everyday world), whereas sexually transmitted diseases which were often construed in *occupational* terms (since they involve regular 'career-like' attendance at the STD clinic). In this respect, it is perhaps significant to note that none of the young people we interviewed differentiated AIDS from other consequences of HIV infection such as Persistent Generalized Lymphadenopathy and AIDS Related Complex. AIDS was almost always seen as a destroyer, not only of the individual concerned, but of relationships between them and other people.

It was rather less easy to anticipate, however, the extent to which young people would operate with *serendipitous* logic in estimating their own risk of acquiring HIV infection and/or AIDS. We were also surprised by the degree of homology we found between *essentialist* understandings of cancer and beliefs about AIDS. These two systems of belief (the serendipitous and the essentialist) may be particularly powerful dis-orienters of official health education intervention within the context of AIDS where many campaigns have stressed in rational terms the avoidable nature of the syndrome. If people are widely perceived as developing AIDS either through 'chance' or 'bad luck', or because it was 'in them' in the first place, the strategies adopted in present campaigns (which by and large make the assumption that people are going to be receptive to notions of risk minimization) may need to be re-thought.

Conclusions

In this chapter we have reported on preliminary findings from a series of in-depth interviews carried out in connection with the project *Young People's Health Knowledge and AIDS*. We have restricted our attention to a consideration of the ways in which young people attending community based youth groups and YTS programmes conceptualized and 'made sense' of HIV infection and AIDS. Subsequently we will report on data collected from young people participating in lesbian and gay youth groups as well as on regional data identifying class, gender and racial differences in lay beliefs about HIV infection and AIDS.

We argued earlier, as we have done elsewhere (Aggleton and Homans, 1987a and 1987b; Aggleton, Homans and Warwick, 1988), that research into lay beliefs about HIV infection and AIDS is important in helping health educationists, policy makers and others anticipate the ways in which people are likely to respond to public information campaigns and health education interventions. This research is also important in allowing us to identify the factors operating to affect personal perceptions of risk. Our findings here suggest that while the young people we have talked to show some understanding and awareness of the ways in which they can minimize their own risk of infection, this knowledge is uneven. In this respect, it is important to recognize that their knowledge parallels that of adults interviewed in studies such as those by Vass (1986), Mills (1987) and Campbell and Waters (1987). It is not that young people are especially 'ignorant' or 'confused' about the issues. Rather, their lay beliefs would seem to be in some respects comparable to those of other sections of the community. It is particularly clear from our preliminary enquiries that mainstream professional explanations of HIV infection and AIDS are at best moderately well understood. Talk of 'the virus' and 'the actual AIDS' would seem to have confused many of those we have spoken to, and young people's continuing belief that there is 'something' which can be easily caught would be appear to have been effectively countered by the efforts that have been made so far to make people more aware of conventional scientific and medical distinctions between HIV infection and AIDS.

In our research we have also been able to identify a variety of lay logics relating to causation. Many of these reaffirm the continuing importance of some of the lay beliefs about health and illness identified by earlier researchers. For example, serendipitous understandings which suggest that whether or not one contracts HIV infection or develops AIDS is largely a matter of chance or bad luck, seem to be closely linked to notions that 'the virus' or 'the actual AIDS' can be easily transmitted. Beliefs like these can serve to undermine the feelings of personal control which young people might otherwise have.[4] Serendipitous theories were generally used when explaining events which might affect interviewees personally, whereas in explaining events affecting others, respondents were more likely to make distinctions between the 'innocent' and 'guilty' victims of diseases, so bringing in notions of personal responsibility.

In a cross-sectional and in-depth study of lay beliefs such as this there is always the danger of presenting an overly homogeneous account of events. The data reported on in this chapter should therefore be seen within the context of ongoing enquiry to identify the varieties of lay beliefs about AIDS and HIV infection that different groups of young people operate with as well as changes within these over time. Future research will undoubtedly add to our understanding of the ways in which race, class, gender, age and sexual preference interact in structuring how young people understand HIV infection and AIDS.

Notes

1   We are grateful to Stuart Watson for helping us identify the importance of the distinction between lay beliefs to do with the immediate 'causes' of AIDS and lay beliefs to do with the syndrome's ultimate origins within the data we have analyzed.
2   It is important to recognize that in this respect Steve's views, like those of many adults, are informed by the view that AIDS is either *contagious* or *infectious* when in reality it is neither. Whilst HIV may be infectious under specific conditions, it is not contagious in the sense that it can be transmitted via touch or objects. AIDS itself is, of course, a medically diagnosed syndrome, being one of the possible consequences of HIV infection. Medically defined syndromes are neither infectious nor contagious.
3   We have placed inverted commas around the term 'victim' in an effort to distance ourselves from discourse of victimatology that is so pervasively used to 'make sense' of HIV infection and AIDS.
4   It is salutory to remember that young people as a whole are systematically denied access to a variety of means by which their own safety and that of others might be enhanced within the context of HIV infection and AIDS. Both their legal status as non-adults and the 'taken for granted assumptions' that inform access (or non-access) to information about safer forms of sexual expression, make them especially vulnerable at the present time.

References

AGGLETON, P. and HOMANS, H. (1987a) *Educating about AIDS — A Discussion Document for Health Education Officers, Community Physicians et al.* Bristol, National Health Service Training Authority.

AGGLETON, P. J. and HOMANS, H. (1987b) 'Teaching AIDS', *Social Science Teacher*, 17, 1, pp. 24–81.

AGGLETON, P. J., HOMANS, H and WARWICK, I. (1988) 'Health education, sexuality and AIDS', paper given at the Xth International Conference on Sociology of Education, Birmingham, to appear in BARTON, L. and WALKER, S. (Eds.) *The Politics of Schooling*, Milton Keynes, Open University Press.

ALTMAN, D. (1986) *AIDS and the New Puritanism*, London, Pluto Press.

ANDERSON, D. (1986) 'Facts that stay concealed', *The Times*, 19 August.

BOLOGNONE, D. and JOHNSON, T. (1986) 'Explanatory models for AIDS' in FIELDMAN, D and JOHNSON, T. (Eds.) *The Social Dimensions of AIDS*, New York, Praeger.

CAMPBELL, M. and WATERS, W. (1987) 'Public knowledge about AIDS increasing', *British Medical Journal*. 294. pp. 892–4.

CLIFT, S. and STEARS, S. (1987) 'A study of students' beliefs and attitudes about AIDS', working paper, Christ Church College, Canterbury.

DiCLEMENTE, R. J., ZORN, J. and TEMOSHOK, L. (1986) 'Adolescents and AIDS: A survey of knowledge, attributes and beliefs about AIDS in San Francisco', *American Journal of Public Health*, 76, 12. pp. 1443–5.

DONOVAN, J. (1986) *We Don't Buy Sickness, It Just Comes*, Aldershot, Gower.

FITZPATRICK, R. (1984) 'Lay concepts of illness' in FITZPATRICK, R. *et al. The experience of Illness*, London, Tavistock.

GRAHAM, H. (1984) *Women, Health and the Family*. Brighton, Wheatsheaf.

Guardian (1986) 'Anderton see AIDS as gays' own fault', 12 December

HART, N. (1985) *The Sociology of Health and Medicine*, Lancashire, Causeway Books.

HELMAN, C (1978) '"Feed a cold, starve a fever": Folk models of infection in an English suburban community and their relation to medical treatment', *Culture, Medicine and Psychiatry*, 2, pp. 107–37.

HERZLICH, C. (1973) *Health and Illness: A Social Psychological Analysis*, New York, Academic Press.

HERZLICH, C. and PIERRET, J. (1986) 'Illness: from causes to meaning' in CURRER, C. and STACEY, M. (Eds.) *Concepts of Health, Illness and Disease*. Leamington Spa. Berg.

HOMANS, H. (1985) 'Discomforts in pregnancy: Traditional remedies and medical prescriptions' in HOMANS, H. (Ed.) *The Sexual Politics of Reproduction*. Aldershot, Gower.

HOMANS, H., AGGLETON, P. J. and WARWICK, I. (1987) *Learning about AIDS — Interim Materials*, London, Health Education Authority/AVERT.

D'HOUTARD, A. and FIELD, M. (1984) 'The image of health: Variations in perception by social class in a French population', *Sociology of Health and Illness*, 6, 1, pp. 30–60.

HUMPHREYS, L. (1970) *Tearoom Trade: Impersonal Sex in Public Places*. Chicago, Aldine.

ILLSLEY, R. *et al* (1977) Review paper in *Health and Health Policy: Perspectives for Research*, report of an advisory panel to the Research Initiatives Board, Social Science Research Council.

JACOBSON, P. (1981) *The Lady Killers: Why Smoking is a Feminist Issue*, London, Pluto Press.

KLEINMAN, A. (1976) 'Concepts and a model for the comparison of medical systems as cultural systems', paper presented to the Theory in Medical Anthropology Conference, National Science Foundation, Washington DC.

MCINTYRE, S. (1986) 'Health and illness' in BURGESS, R. (Ed.) *Key Variables in Social Investigation*, London, Routledge and Kegan Paul.

MCKEOWN, T. (1979) *The Role of Medicine*, Oxford, Basil Blackwell.

MILLS, S. *et al* (1987) 'Attitudes and trends: Public perceptions of AIDS', *Focus — A Review of AIDS Research*, 2, 1, pp. 1–3.

PATTON, C (1985) *Sex and Germs*, Boston, MA, South End Press.

PILL, R. and SCOTT, N. (1982) 'Concepts of illness causation and responsibility:

Some preliminary data from a sample of working class mothers', *Social Science and Medicine*, 16, pp. 13–51.

REISS, A. J. (1961) 'The social integration of queers and peers', *Social Problems*, 9, pp. 102–19.

SEABROOK, J. (1973) *The Underprivileged: A Hundred Years of Family Life and Tradition in a Working Class Street*, Harmondsworth, Penguin Books.

SEARLE, J. (1987) 'Knowledge, attitudes and behaviour of health professionals in relation to AIDS', *Lancet*, i, pp. 26–8.

SONTAG, S. (1979) *Illness as Metaphor*, New York, Vintage Books.

Times (1984) Editorial, 21 November.

UNSCHULD, P. (1986) 'The conceptual determination of individual and collective experiences of illness' in CURRER, C. and STACEY, M. (Eds.) *Concepts of Health, Disease and Illness*, Leamington Spa, Berg.

VASS, A. (1986) *A Plague In Us*, Cambridge, Venus Academica.

WATNEY, S. (1987) 'AIDS, "moral panic" theory and homophobia', Chapter 3 in this volume.

WEINBERG, T. (1983) *Gay Men, Gay Selves*, New York, Irvington.

WELLINGS, K. (1987) 'Perceptions of risk: Media treatments of AIDS', chapter 5 in this volume.

WORLD HEALTH ORGANISATION (1946) *Constitution of First People*, WHO, Geneva.

ZOLA, I. (1966) 'Culture and symptoms — An analysis of patients' presenting complaints', *American Sociological Review*, 31, pp. 615–30.

7
The Numbers Game — Gay Lifestyles, Epidemiology of Aids and Social Science

Tony Coxon

In recent years, medical science has provided us with considerable insight into the nature and consequences of Human Immunodeficiency Virus (HIV) infection and AIDS. Medical scientists and epidemiologists have also attempted to predict or model the extent to which HIV infection may become more prevalent over the next few years. In order to make these predictions, mathematical models are frequently constructed out of the factors or parameters which are believed to influence the development of a particular epidemic. Of particular importance within the modelling of HIV infection are parameters which identify both the *number of sexual partners* an individual has and *particular sexual acts* (primarily anal intercourse) as critical factors affecting the rate of transmission of HIV.

But social science too is needed in order to understand the role played by particular patterns of sexual behaviour in the epidemiology of HIV infection. There are good reasons to suppose that epidemiological analyses which take at face value the self-reports which individuals give concerning the frequency and types of sexual acts they participate in may be seriously flawed in the predictions they make. The social context in which data is collected as well as expectancies about the uses to which it is to be put both influence the reliability and validity of the self-reports that people give.

In this chapter, I will try to identify some of the methodological, technical and substantive factors which interact in the collection of data relating to male gay behaviour. An attempt will also be made to explore the implications of these issues for efforts to predict the rate at which HIV infection may spread. In particular, attention will be focussed on two crucial parameters in epidemiological studies of AIDS — the number of sexual partners and the prevalence of receptive anal intercourse. In exploring the issues associated with making reliable and valid estimates of these forms of sexual behaviour, reference will be made to research investigating changes in sexual behaviour of gay men within the context of AIDS. This project, Project Sigma — *A longitudinal study of the sexual behaviour of homosexual men under the impact of AIDS* — is concerned to investigate the current sexual lifestyles of gay and bisexual/married men. By interviewing respondents in this study at six month intervals and by asking them to keep detailed sexual diaries in between these interview points, it is possible o detect and evaluate changes in their sexual and related behaviour.

Medicine and Social Science

Many issues to do with AIDS, HIV infection, sero-positivity and infectivity are by their very nature medically defined. But being HIV antibody positive or being diagnosed as having AIDS is more than simply a medical matter, since these conditions profoundly affect people, their relationships and lives. The consequences of HIV infection can therefore be as serious socially and economically as they can be in medical terms. The competences required to study these latter aspects are not medical. Indeed an analysis of the psychological, sociological and economic aspects of HIV infection and AIDS may even be hindered by medical attitudes and orientations since here the issues are of a different order to those usually encountered in medical practice.

But this is not simply a plea merely for a fuller consideration of the social *consequences* of HIV infection and AIDS. In response to the claim made by many doctors that 'laypeople' are unable to contribute directly to purely medical matters, it may be important to point out that, equally, medical scientists and clinicians rarely possess the competence necessary to fully understand social aspects of their human data — competences which stem primarily from training within the social sciences.

Three interdisciplinary and professional rivalries would not be so serious if they did not have consequences for determining priorities in the funding of AIDS-related research. The most obvious example of this can be found in health education and AIDS. It is ironic that whilst enormous effort and cost is given to ensuring that drugs and vaccines are monitored and evaluated, it is assumed that health education to change sexual behaviour needs no corresponding investment. Only after considerable pressure have self-help groups such as the Terrence Higgins Trust and Body Positive received any government funding, and then the amount they have received has been small in comparison to their needs and activities. People have become accustomed to government action which is purely responsive to crises and which enthrones financial self-help as a prime virtue. But the irony is that even on these terms many aspects of present policy are counter-productive. Lack of funding now not simply means more deaths, but also unnecessary suffering and grossly more expensive health care costs in the future.

However, brave claims about the value of social science analysis with respect to AIDS are not enough. We need to demonstrate how medical issues can be illuminated by social science and how an ignorance of social science may impede or even nullify medical findings. In those aspects of medical science in particular which aim to develop theory from the self-reports which people give about their own behaviour (and this includes activities as diverse as taking clinical life-histories and obtaining information on prevalence of certain behaviours, in addition to more obvious areas like medical counselling), approaches to data collection and analysis which ignore sociologically relevant insights are simply deficient; these areas *need* social science input, if they are to be scientifically credible.

HIV Infection, Epidemiology and AIDS

Nowhere is this need more obvious and important than in epidemiological studies, dependent as they are on behavioural observation, report and information. In the case of the epidemiology of AIDS in particular, we are dealing with a domain that is only slightly less delicate to enquire into than income. For much of the relevant data will of necessity relate to groups that are socially stigmatized (intravenous drug users, prostitutes, gay and bisexual men) and to sexual activities that are personal, sometimes illegal and often socially invisible. Taken together these issues are likely to make us question the reliability and validity of conventional data-collection procedures, and manifestly require the use of sophisticated research skills.

Instead of this, in most epidemiological studies of HIV infection, sexual behaviour and AIDS we typically find a heavy reliance on data collected in *clinical settings*, combined with an uncritical willingness to extrapolate from dubious American studies of sexual behaviour conducted within from the pre-AIDS era. In this chapter I do not intend to discuss in any detail the distortions which can be introduced into our understandings of sexual behaviour by inappropriate sampling techniques nor by the social dynamics of the interview situation. Nevertheless, we need to recognize that sexual behavioural studies of those who already have a history of sexually transmitted disease (a persistent and clearly powerful co-factor in the etiology of AIDS) are unlikely to provide an unbiased picture of the behaviour of the entire at-risk population. Furthermore, being interviewed within the medical context of a clinic, by an interviewer who may be far from informed and possibly homophobic, augurs ill for truth-telling.

Reliability and Self-report Data

More disturbing in many ways is the clear and repeated evidence from research which suggests that *in general* the reliability of data gathered in such studies of sexual behaviour may be low (Coxon, 1986a; McManus and McEvoy, 1985). This is especially true of the very detailed information necessary for sophisticated epidemiological modelling. The main points concerning this lack of reliability can be summarized schematically as follows.

First, we rely on people's willingness to *report* sexual behaviour to *infer* information about its quality and quantity. This raises serious problems concerning the reliability of the estimates that people may give. Very few studies have attempted to triangulate upon the 'same' sexual events in order to assess the reliability of the claims that one of the parties involved may make. In our own work exploring the dynamics of gay behaviour we have used diary methods to examine the sexual practices of our respondents. On occasions where both sexual partners have been project subjects (either as a couple or contingently) and have completed daily sexual diaries, it has been possible to study triangulated accounts of these 'same' events. Preliminary findings concerning the reliability of data collected by this method suggests that the convergence between accounts is usually surprisingly good so long as the events concerned are recorded soon after their occurrence and the people reporting these are well-motivated and accept the guarantees of confidentiality and anonymity they have been given.

Second, studies of the *reliability* of self-reports of sexual behaviour show that in general, the retrospective recall of information tends to be selective, ordinally distorted and unreliable. Research which attempts to identify when respondents *first* gained particular sexual experiences is likely to show the same biases. However, our research suggests that when it comes to investigating more recent events, it is possible to increase the reliability of the data by repeatedly asking the same questions or by implying them at several points in the course of the same interview. In linear regression analyses of respondents' estimates of their reported daily behaviour, however, we find systematic individual differences both in overall accuracy and in distortion. Knowing this, individual accounts can be compared; without it, individual comparisons can be highly misleading.

Third, in trying to track the detail and sequencing of sexual behaviour, time-lapse is also an important factor to take into account in assessing the reliability (in the test-retest sense) of the data. The further back in time an event occurred, the less reliable people's reports become. In general, our research seems to suggest that people seem generally incapable of recalling accurately what happened a fortnight ago, let alone before this.

On these three sets of grounds we should be critical of the reliability of data emanating from routine inventories of sexual behaviour collected in a busy clinic for the treatment of sexually transmitted diseases. When this same data is subsequently used to provide parameter estimates of the frequency and nature of particular sexual acts for use in modelling the spread of infection within a particular population, there are grounds for further concern.

Reliably Estimating the Number of Sexual Partners

Nowhere are the consequences of low-quality data-collection more important than in assessing the reliability (and hence the validity) of the responses given to apparently innocuous questions about the 'number of partners' an individual may have had. On *a priori* grounds it might be imagined that those who are sexually exclusive/monogamous would have no difficulty answering such a question, those who have multiple (regular) partners might have some, and that the rest (the promiscuous, the sluts or the sexual athletes according to one's point of view) might have a great deal. In fact two quite different issues are intertwined here: *accuracy of recall* on the one hand and *definitional problems* relating to what is meant by the term 'sexual partner' on the other.

Problems to do with accuracy of recall are easier to deal with, since they relate to the issues of reliability earlier discussed. In recalling sexual encounters, there certainly seems to be a recency effect (people remember best what has happened in the immediate past), but from our research the accuracy of their recall also depends on how varied a person's sex-life is and how large or significant a fraction of it is comprised of one-off contacts. As in the case of reliability of reported sexual acts, we have been able in our work to check the estimates our respondents give of the number of sexual contacts they have against the actual number they record in their sexual diaries. When we do this, however, the news is not good since estimates of the number of partners (and hence of the rate of change in partners) seem to be *least* dependable when people make reference to their non-regular partners. Since their sexual behaviour is also least predictable for such contacts, and their partner's antibody status is less likely to be known (and as there is a higher chance of alcohol and/or drugs being involved), there are important consequences here for attempts to estimate epidemiological parameters from such data. This is to put on one side entirely the issue of health risks.

But this is not all. If we look more closely at some of the questionnaires that have been to gain estimates of the number of sexual partners that gay men attending clinics for the treatment of sexually transmitted diseases may have had, we find that in many cases answers to questions about the 'number of partners' could not be given in an openended way. Rather, subjects are often provided with fixed pre-supplied categories. Significantly, these categories are rarely of equal-intervals, but follow an implicit power relation: small intervals at the least frequent end of the scale, working up to large ones at the most frequent end. They thus produce *as an artefact* the evidence of 'promiscuity' so often uncritically quoted in the medical and other press (figure 1).

There are good grounds therefore to be suspicious on technical grounds of the reliability and validity of data collected in clinic situations concerning the number of sexual partners an individual has had. But there are other important issues here to do with cognitive and socio-semantic matters.

Figure 1: Questions asked during a recent survey of male homosexual behaviour

18 How many different male sexual partners have you had in the past year?

None	☐
Less than 5	☐
6–50	☐
51–100	☐
101–500	☐
501–1,000	☐
1000 or more	☐

19 How many different male sexual partners have you had in your lifetime?

None	☐
Less than 5	☐
6–50	☐
51–100	☐
101–500	☐
501–1000	☐
1001–2500	☐
2501–5000	☐
5001–10,000	☐
10,000 or more	☐

Even were we to provide potential respondents with an open-ended or evenly graduated scale of categories, it is important to know how much confidence the respondent gives to the estimate. In this respect, it is surprising how often crucial prefatory comments which indicate that respondents are unsure about the estimates they are about to make can be ignored in recording and analyzing the data. Bell and Weinberg (1978) are virtually unique in asking their interviewers to find out how respondents arrived at their estimated numbers of sexual partners by providing them with the following coded alternatives: 'Rough guess/grossing up/reasonably precise number/exact number'.

Again, not surprisingly, we find that the reliability of these estimates is negatively associated with stated number of partners. There are exceptions: some people appear to carry around a mental diary which they can quote from *ad libitum*, and others clearly set themselves targets. But however celebrated the latter category of person may be in the world of literature, they tend to be rare in practice. In our research, we have been struck with how often a strategy of 'grossing up' is used for estimating anything over a week. As we have found for reported sexual behaviour, the week is usually the critical period of time which can be recalled quite well. When asked to provide estimates over a longer period, subjects will typically 'multiply up' their weekly figure. To the extent that this is true, what one gets in response to such questions is *not* a report on a longer period, but an extrapolation from one (perhaps atypical) week. It may well be that the responses people also give to questions about changes in their sexual behaviour over the last *n* weeks or months have exactly the same shortcomings.

But the most critical issue is: what do people actually mean when they talk of a 'sexual partner'? (and, for that matter, what do researchers?). Without this knowledge we have no basis to make inter-individual comparisons. In particular, if a respondent's conception of a 'sexual partner' does not conform to the researcher's idea of what is meant by this term, then data collection and subsequent analysis will at best be biased and at worst meaningless.

In our own longitudinal studies of the sexual behaviour of gay men, we initially adopted as a tentative working definition of a 'sexual partner' — 'anyone with whom you had any form of sexual experience except wanking when no-one came' — only to find that this failed to do justice to the range of definitions with which our respondents operated. Subsequent work has shown the variety of respondents' definitions to be truly immense. At one extreme may be the man who enjoys sado-masochism (S & M) and who counts as any 'sexual partner' any other man who manifests an erection in an S & M scene. At the other may be men who only count as 'sexual partners' those with whom they have had anal intercourse to the point of orgasm. Between these two extremes lie many other variations. In the light of this, in studies attempting to gain reliable estimates of sexual behaviour, respondents and researchers need to explore carefully and systematically what each other mean when they talk of 'sexual partners' and 'sexual acts'.

Modelling the Transmission of HIV Infection

How are these points relevant to the broader medical and sociological referred to earlier in this chapter? Given what we currently know about the processes involved in HIV transmission, epidemiological modelling of the likely spread of infection is crucially dependent on the availability of reliable and valid estimates of the prevalence of those acts most intimately connected with viral transmission. Two such parameters are *the number of sexual partners* an individual has and the extent to which *receptive anal intercourse* is practised. For reasons already discussed, reliable and valid estimates of these two parameters will be difficult, if not impossible, to come by using conventional data collection procedures.

But there are other problems too. Modelling the spread of an epidemic such as HIV infection (amongst gay men at least) may be further complicated by the fact that there is an asymmetry of partner exchange rates amongst gay men. Whereas within the heterosexual context the *rates* of partner exchange are equal between men and women, in the case of homosexual populations this is not so because gay men engage in anally insertive and anally receptive acts with different and unequal rates of partner exchange for each of these acts. It would be simpler from the point of view of epidemiological modelling if those engaging in anal intercourse would adopt a consistent role — and indeed for some time epidemiological models assumed that they did. The picture is further complicated by the fact that these two forms of sexual behaviour are associated with considerably different risks of infection. Knox (1986) for example has recently claimed that, 'about 95 per cent of all known AIDS-infected homosexual and bisexual men are reported as A(nally) R(eceptive)'. Whilst statements like these are important in identifying the sexual acts which are particularly dangerous insofar as the transmission of HIV is concerned, they effectually presuppose that gay and bisexual men adopt a consistent role in anal intercourse: a claim which needs further consideration.

Kinds of Homosexual or Types of Sexual Behaviour?

Effective epidemiological modelling of HIV infection crucially depends on information about sexual behaviour obtained from *non-clinical populations*. Until very recently this information has been derived from what elsewhere I have identified as 'a willingness to conjure information out of thin air or by extrapolation from dubious American studies of the pre-AIDS era' (Coxon, 1986b). In this context it may be salutory to think about an incident some months ago when within the space of the same week two eminent medical experts proclaimed, and with no qualification, that 'the' fraction of homosexuals who were 'passive' was 90 per cent in one case and 50 per cent in the other. It can firmly be said that there are *no* reliable estimates of this sort currently available for Britain, not least because to obtain them we would have to pre-suppose that amongst gay men, behaviour is thus segregated. Certainly preliminary data from our own research suggests that a far higher fraction of men engage in both of these practices (but with different rates of partner exchange for each of them) than restrict themselves to one.

In obtaining estimates of key parameters within their epidemiological models, Knox and others rely primarily on studies by Kinsey (1948) and on Gagnon and Simon (1974) for their data. There are problems with this data however since not only was it collected some time ago but within a cultural context very different to that of modern Britain. Unfortunately, the estimates given for the prevalance of certain forms of sexual behaviour in these studies have a tendency to become accepted 'truths' or 'facts'. As an example of this, we can consider Knox's (1986) recent claim (taken accurately, it should be stressed from Gagnon and Simon's work) that, 'the AP ("active") homosexuals are many times (for example × 20) as promiscuous as the AR ("passive") homosexuals, and therefore much less (for example, × 0.05) frequent in this sub-population (of homosexuals)' (p. 167).

Now the empirical basis for Gagnon and Simon's original claim is tenuous to say the least, being based on estimates obtained from non-representative samples even within the American context. But here we can see what was originally a provisional estimate becoming part of received wisdom — being written into an epidemiological model as a key parameter predicting future patterns of HIV infection in Britain. Given our general lack of knowledge concerning the prevalence of particular types of sexual practices amongst members of non-clinical populations in Britain it is hard at present to counter such claims empirically but data from the our research on Project Sigma may in time allow this.

But where do such dangerously misleading images and understandings of male homosexual behaviour come from? Their recent origins can be traced back to psychiatric explanations which seek to understand this behaviour in terms of 'conventional' heterosexual practices. At their crudest, such theories argued that all gay men simply identified with the female gender. Subsequent accounts identified two exclusive types: the socially visible 'effeminate passive' homosexual and the (unseen) 'dominant active' homosexual.

Following Bieber's *et al* (1962) work in the early 1960s, these two types of homosexual men came to be equated with two types of sexual behaviour. It was they who coined the terms 'insector' and 'insertee' to reflect this supposedly fundamental difference in sexual activity. Significantly of course the data which allow such claims to be made derive from clinical samples. It is important to recognize though that views like these were challenged by more sensitive observers at the time they were made. Westwood (1960), for example, was already insisting that all homosexual men could not be typified as exclusively active or passive and pointed out that a significant number of them regularly interchanged roles. These views were subsequently echoed in Harry and DeVall's (1978) work.

Elsewhere I have argued that we should abandon the notion that gay men are predominantly anything, and adopt instead the more realistic assumption that gay males engage in a range of both types of behaviour (Coxon, 1986a and 1986b). This means abandoning the insertor/ee and active/passive typing of *people*, to reserve this distincting only for *acts*. Which of these acts individuals engage in depends critically upon the situation and the type of relationship they are in. In order to develop more sophisticated epidemiological models relating to HIV infection we need to know precisely what differentiates sexual behaviour in these various contexts.

Interaction Between the Number of Partners and Types of Sexual Acts

But that is not the end of the matter. As was pointed out earlier, epidemiological models quite rightly identify as key parameters affecting HIV transmission, anal intercourse and rates of change of partners. But until recently many have failed to explore the crucial role of interaction between these two variables in determining the relative 'safety' of particular sexual acts. Recent research by Van Grienfven *et al* (1986) in the Netherlands has begun to investigate some of the behavioural factors discriminating between those who do and those who do not acquire HIV infection following particular patterns of sexual activity. The results are striking. Not just for anal intercourse, but *in general*, it is the *interaction* of the particular sex act and the number of partners (NP) that does the discriminating between whether or not a person becomes HIV infected, rather than either factor separately (figure 2).

Shown as an operating characteristic, it is clear that 'number of partners' accelerates in different ways depending on the risk of the behaviour concerned. Sometimes, indeed usually, it does this linearly with a varying slope. However, in the case of anally receptive (AR) acts it does this as a strong power function. The difference between $AR \times NP$ and $AP \times = NP$ here is quite striking.

Figure 2: *HIV seropositivity, number of sexual partners and sexual acts*

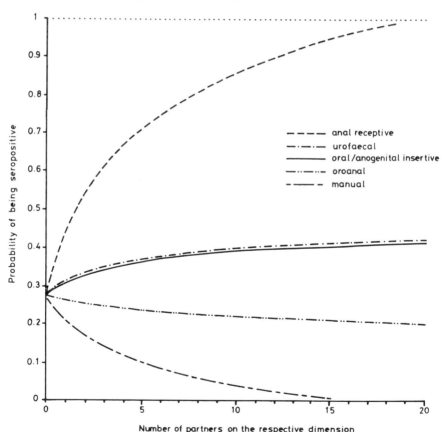

Source: Van Grienfven *et al* (1986).

For those involved in health education there may be a number of lessons to learn from this data. Perhaps future health education messages should not simply urge gay men to use condoms when having anal sex, but should say quite plainly, 'If you are fucked, you are at by far the greatest risk, and this risk increases dramatically with every different partner'.

Conclusions

In this chapter I have tried to do two things. First, efforts have been made to identify some of the social factors influencing the reliability and validity of data relating to gay male practices. I have been critical of the inferences clinicians and others have drawn from research based on clinical samples of gay men, and have argued that further enquiry is needed to identify the nature and variability of gay male practice. Data from Project Sigma — *A longitudinal study of the sexual behaviour of homosexual men under the impact of AIDS* — may in time provide this.

Second, I have tried to identify some of the problems inherent in the epidemiological modelling of HIV infection. Until we have reliable and valid estimates of various kinds of sexual behaviour it would seem likely that we shall continue to have difficulty in making predictions about the possible spread of infection and in devising health education programmes based upon sound knowledge about the relative 'safety' of particular sexual practices.

References

BELL, A. P. and WEINBERG, M. (1978) *Homosexualities: A Study of Diversity Among Men and Women*, New York, Simon and Schuster.

BIEBER, I. *et al*, (1962) *Homosexuality: A Psychoanalytic Study*, New York, Basic Books.

COXON, A. P. M. (1986a) *Report on Pilot Study: Project on Sexual Lifestyles of Non-heterosexual Males*, Cardiff, SRU

COXON, A. P. M. (1986b) '*It all depends ... the impact of context on patterns of homosexual behaviour*', paper given at Medical Sociology Conference, University of York.

GAGNON, J. H. and SIMON, W. (1974) *Sexual Conduct: The Social Sources of Human Sexuality*, Chicago, Aldine.

HARRY, J. and DEVALL, W. B. (1978) *The Social Organization of Gay Males*, New York, Praeger.

KNOX, E. (1986) 'A transmission model for AIDS', *European Journal of Epidemiology*. 2, 3, pp. 165–77.

McMANUS, T. J. and McEVOY, M. (1985) A preliminary study of some aspects of male homosexual behaviour in the United Kingdom, London, Kings College Hospital. Submitted for publication.

WESTWOOD, G. (1960) *A Minority: A Report on the Life of the Male Homosexual in Great Britain*, London, Longmans

VAN GRIENFVEN, G. J., TIELEMAN, R. A. P. and GOLDSMIT, J. (1986) 'Prevalence of LAV/HTLV III antibodies in relation to lifestyle characteristics in homosexual men in the Netherlands', paper presented at the International Conference on AIDS, Paris, June.

8
AIDS — A Trade Union Issue

Hugh Robertson

In this chapter I intend to explore why HIV infection and AIDS is an issue for the British trade union movement by identifying some of the ways in which different trade unions have responded to AIDS so far. I will focus in particular on the rather different factors which have led two major trade unions to make very different responses to AIDS and AIDS-related issues. Finally, I hope to show that the trade union movement could play a greater role in tackling the issues raised by HIV infection and AIDS than it has done so far.

Initially, however, it is important to put discussion of these issues in context. Trade unions are far from peripheral to any debate concerning the social aspects of AIDS. The British trade union movement plays a unique role in British society. Proportionately it is the largest and strongest trade union movement in the non-communist world. Despite assaults on trade union rights over the last seven years, mass unemployment and the defeat of the miners' strike, the trade unions are still a major social force, with in excess of ten million members and negotiating rights in most major industries and services. They have also, to some extent, been responsible for much of the progressive social change that has occurred over the last century.

What therefore are the implications of AIDS for this movement? In this chapter four separate, but interconnected, areas of trade union interest will be discussed. These concern conditions of service, health and safety at work, equal opportunities, and National Health Service resource provision.

Conditions of Service

Issues relating to conditions of service are those matters which arise directly in connection with a person's employment with an employer. The most obvious problem in this area arises when the employer finds out a worker has been diagnosed as having AIDS or as HIV antibody positive. On these occasions, and in spite of recent advice from the Department of Employment to the contrary, [1] it is still likely that an employer will attempt to suspend or dismiss the person concerned. Other employers have in the past removed HIV antibody positive people from working with members of the public. [2]

This policy has, on occasion, been extended to known gay men, and there is every possibility that unless it is resisted, it may in future be extended to haemophiliacs and known or suspected intravenous drug users. In one incident of this type an employee was dismissed on the grounds that the employer had eczema and therefore believed he was at risk from having a gay man working in the same office as him, despite there being no evidence that the gay man had ever been exposed to the HIV virus. [3] Such actions are clearly irresponsible since not only is the risk of transmission at work minimal if reasonable precautions are taken, but it is important for people with AIDS, or who are HIV antibody positive, to be encouraged to work if they so wish.

Apart from direct discrimination against people currently in employment, there is the related issue of screening potential employees by such means as insisting that job applicants deemed to be in a 'high risk' group should be tested for antibodies to HIV before being admitted into company or local authority pension schemes. [4] There have even been cases of employers testing samples of blood taken for other purposes without telling the employee concerned. Additionally, there is a need for time off and sick leave agreements to cater for the needs of people with AIDS or AIDS related illnesses, and to provide additional support for those who are caring for people with AIDS.

Health and Safety at Work

Although HIV infection presents no significant occupational hazard, many workers quite erroneously perceive this to be the case. In view of the way in which AIDS has been presented in the popular press, it is hardly surprising that many people are deeply concerned about the possibility of contacting AIDS through their employment.

Advice for medical staff was first issued by the Advisory Committee on Dangerous Pathogens (ACDP) in December 1984, and these guidelines have been revised since then. They outline measures which should be taken by health authorities to ensure that nursing, medical and other staff who may come into direct contact with the virus should be protected from possible infection. It is important to recognize, however, that these guidelines have been issued at a time when public sector health service provision in Britain is being starved of funding, and health and safety is often given low priority by hospital management. In addition, these guidelines have not been widely circulated within the NHS and are written in a style which is clearly aimed at hospital administrators and medical staff. Little has so far been produced in an easily understandable form for general circulation to all NHS staff, and within our hospitals many workers who have day-to-day contact with people with AIDS have no informed knowledge either of what AIDS is or how it is transmitted. Related to this are as yet unreconciled debates about whether staff should be informed if they are dealing with people with HIV infection and/or AIDS, and about how hospitals are going to deal with the issue of confidentiality.

Most of the concern over health and safety has, however, been voiced by non-NHS workers. These include social workers, cleaners, firefighters, home-helps, teachers, and even telephone engineers, who at one point refused to repair the telephones of London lesbian and gay switchboard for fear of contracting AIDS.[5]

In some instances, this concern may be little more than direct homophobia masquerading under the guise of fear of AIDS, but in most cases it is a result of a lack of information and advice from employers. Where health and safety at work issues have been fully discussed with those workers, these problems have often been resolved.

However it is not just a question of reassuring workers like home-helps and cleaners. In many of the so-called 'caring professions', workers are dealing directly with soiled linen, blood spillage, vomit and the disposal of waste, and need to be given advice on the common sense precautions that should be taken, not just to avoid HIV infection, but the more likely infection by other blood-borne viruses. In most occupations, employers have not provided information about these precautions.

One additional area where health and safety arguments have been aired is, of course, where members are working with other workers who have AIDS or are HIV antibody positive. There are examples of trade union members refusing to work with such people or insisting that they be barred from using canteens and other communal facilities.[6] Incidents of this type have in the past generally been tackled after the problem has arisen rather than proactively by proper programmes of AIDS education before they have a chance to occur.

Equal Opportunities

Although health and safety at work is the area which has elicited the most sustained response from trade unions, it is in the field of equal opportunities that AIDS has already had the most impact. In recent years there has been a rising tide of homophobia within the workplace as the spread of AIDS has been closely identified with gay men and, by implication, lesbians. The limited work that has been done by trade unions in fighting for lesbian and gay rights, culminating in the passing of a strong and positive resolution at the 1985 TUC conference, has been grossly undermined by the inaccurate and sensationalist media reporting of AIDS. Gay activists within the trade union movement now find themselves under considerable pressure, not just from the personal threat that HIV infection and AIDS poses, but from their own work colleagues.

In many work environments, homophobia, disguised as fear of AIDS, is becoming increasingly respectable. In the past homosexuality itself has been seen as contagious. This, combined with media portrayals of gay men as weak and irresponsible, has led many to identify gay men as the cause, rather than the first to suffer from AIDS. In consequence, within the context of AIDS, gay men are frequently denied the care, compassion and understanding which may be given to other more 'innocent' victims of infection (such as babies, the female partners of bisexual men and grandmothers). We now have the media parading the concept of a virus as having a morality. The failure of the trade union movement to tackle homophobia in a consistent and positive way has helped allow this prejudice to develop — a situation which some employers have not been slow to exploit.

It is not appropriate here to chronicle the cases of workers who have been sacked, refused promotion, moved from dealing with the public, or ostracized by their colleagues solely for being gay. Few who read the gay press can be unaware of these events. Suffice it to say that in every workplace where there are lesbians and gay men who are open about their sexuality, there is increased prejudice against them under the guise of fear of AIDS. It is impossible to assess how much of the intensifying homophobia results from members believing the content of ill-informed articles they have read in newspapers, and how much is just a smokescreen for bigotry. But whatever the reason, the real tragedy is that increasing numbers of lesbians and gay men are being prevented from coming out at work by the increasingly hostile climate in which they find themselves.

In the USA and France the media's wrath has also been strongly directed against black people in identifying them with the spread of AIDS. Here in Britain, Conservative politicians too have demanded that entrants to Britain from some African countries be screened for antibodies to the HIV virus.[7] In addition, leaflets have been circulated in London by Right Wing and Fascist groups warning white women that they risk AIDS if the sleep with black men. The racism which AIDS is bringing to the fore is not only insidious, it is also potentially divisive, setting one minority group against another. Issues of racism which are connected with AIDS have not yet been adequently challenged by either trade unions themselves or the lesbian and gay groups within the trade union movement.

Finally, in the area of equal opportunities there is another aspect of prejudice which should be mentioned. This is prejudice about disease itself — especially about disease which is strongly identified with death, and a slow painful death at that. This is a new aspect of prejudice for the trade union movement to deal with, and one which is compounded by most people's belief that they personally are safe from infection, and that those with AIDS are responsible for their own illness.

National Health Service Resource Provision

The fourth aspect of HIV infection and AIDS of relevance to trade union activity is the issue of public sector health service resources. Despite the comparatively low incidence of AIDS in Britain, compared with, say, the United States, the pressure which HIV-related illness is going to place on the National Health Service, and to a lesser extent on local authorities, is going to be considerable.

At the moment the cost of caring for a person with AIDS is put at around £25,000. As we develop more effective methods of tackling either HIV infection itself or the opportunistic infections associated with AIDS, the length of treatment will be greater, and so the cost per patient will increase. This, however, covers only part of the cost of health service provision. Additionally, there will be the expense of intervening with respect to other as yet only partially understood consequences of HIV infection (such as pre-senile dementia), the cost of upgrading hospital facilities, the cost of HIV antibody (and in time antigen) testing, the cost of HIV-related counselling, of staff training, of heat treatment for blood products and of screening all blood donations. The combined expense of additional health service provision such as this is likely to be substantial. Over and above this there is the urgent need for increased expenditure with respect to effective programmes of targetted health education (seen by many as the key to controlling the further spread of HIV infection), and into basic research.

In a situation where health service provision is already badly over-stretched, where will these additional resources be found? Matters are further complicated by the fact that over three-quarters of all presently diagnosed AIDS cases are being treated by the four Thames Regional Health Authorities. Yet these are the same authorities which have suffered the most serious cutbacks as part of recent resource re-distribution programme within the National Health Service. Of the four London hospitals with the highest number of AIDS patients, two have already been forced to merge several of their services, including the casualty department, and one has shut a number of wards which housed isolation facilities. One London Health Authority, Bloomsbury, had to find almost £1 million of additional money in 1985/86 to cover the cost of in-patient, out-patient and pathology services relating to HIV infection and AIDS. In the same year, North Kensington required over £½ million of additional money. These are *Area* Health Authorities within the four Thames Regional Health Authorities already referred to, yet during that year the government made available only £680,000 in new resources to all four of these. The rest of the money had to be found from within existing budgets. That can only mean cuts in services and cuts in jobs.

In addition, the cost to the Blood Transfusion Service of screening blood donations was £3 million in the first year. No new funding for this has been provided.

Where the government has made extra resources available has been via the package of £38 million given to the Blood Products Laboratory to ensure Britain is self-sufficient in blood products. That much needed money had already been withheld for a number of years, and was only granted when it was recognized that there was a considerable risk of HIV infection spreading to the heterosexual community through imported blood products originating in the United States.

At the same time as the present government has forced health authorities to divert money from other areas of patient care, it has pushed through further privatization within the National Health Service itself. This has created additional problems associated with the education and training of workers who are not directly employed by Health Authorities, and for maintaining adequate levels of care for patients and working conditions for staff. The poor pay, falling standards of hygiene and repair, high levels of staff turnover, and poor staff morale which inevitably follow privatization all make such problems worse.

Trade Union Responses

Having identified so far some of the AIDS-related issues currently facing the British trade union movement, it is now appropriate to look at some of the responses which have been made.

Of the ninety two trade unions affiliated to the Trades Union Congress (TUC) just under a third are known to have issued some form of advice or information about AIDS. This has ranged from very comprehensive and detailed guidance relating to members' concerns to a letter grudgingly printed in the Union journal.[8] However, of the ten largest trade unions, which between them account for over 65 per cent of the TUC's membership, the picture is slightly better with all but one having responded to the challenge posed by AIDS in one way or another. Even the TUC itself, which is not always quick to react to a situation, issued a report to affiliates in August 1985.

As might be expected, the health service unions have issued the most detailed advice to their members. Most of this has concentrated on giving guidance on the health and safety aspects of HIV infection and AIDS. A number of craft trade unions have also produced very detailed information for workers in particular industries.

The most comprehensive and detailed policies relating to HIV infection and AIDS have been developed by the larger manual and white-collar unions such as Transport and General Workers' Union (TGWU), the National Union of Public Employees (NUPE), the National Association of Local Government Officers (NALGO) and the General Municipal Boilermakers and Allied Trades Union (GMBATU), while the National Union of Journalists (NUJ), not surprisingly, has concentrated on trying to rectify the media bias by issuing very welcome guidelines to journalists.

Unfortunately some trade unions have taken a more sensationalist stand on AIDS, or have used AIDS as a means by which to settle other grievances. These include the Prison Officer's Association (POA), and the Fire Brigades Union (FBU). Their actions should, however, be seen in context. Both the above cases arose shortly after the death in January 1985 of a prison chaplain diagnosed with AIDS, and at a time when media attention on the disease was at its peak. The POA in particular received a lot of publicity when one of its local representatives threatened to lock gay prisoners in their cells, and not admit any further prisoners. This action was not in accordance with the POA's national position, which was to raise concern over the effects of overcrowding in prisons, the lack of protective clothing, and the failure to provide staff with adequate information on HIV infection and AIDS.

The FBU's position was even more distorted. For some time prior to 1985, the FBU had been calling for the issue of small plastic tubes for use in artificial resuscitation. These tubes cost about 90p each. This equipment had originally been requested to avoid union members becoming infected by blood borne viruses such as Hepatitis B, but this request had been refused by the Home Office. When the FBU mentioned AIDS as one of the reasons for wanting this equipment, its actions were widely interpreted by the popular press as indicating that firefighters were threatening not to give the kiss of life to gay men involved in road accidents. No such threat was ever made, and the FBU's position on AIDS has been relatively positive.

Looking at trade union responses in this way is, however, of limited value for a variety of reasons. First, many of the unions which have produced a detailed policy have failed to effectively communicate that policy to its members. Second, it is impossible to judge a union's response in isolation from the structure and membership of that union, and the climate in which the policy was drawn up. Third, looking at its policies alone does not tell us much about how a particular union is likely to respond to individual cases. Many trade unions which have excellent policies on paper have failed to support individual workers, whilst other unions which may perhaps have no official policy on AIDS have proved to be very supportive when approached by their members for assistance.

Two Styles of Trade Union Response

In order to illustrate how particular policies are arrived at, it is useful to look in detail at the recent actions of two different trade unions with a similar sized membership. Both of these provide models for the broader trade union movement in terms of how they have reacted to the problems raised by AIDS. The two unions concerned are NUPE and NALGO.

NUPE is a public service union with around 700,000 members. A majority of its members are low-paid manual workers and over 150,000 of them work in the National Health Service. Affiliated to the Labour Party, NUPE has a long history of struggle against cutbacks and low pay, and of campaigning for the development of public service provision. Two-thirds of its members are women.

NALGO on the other hand is a white-collar public service union with over 750,000 members covering all aspects of non-manual work. Most of its members work in local government, but it has a similar number of members working in the NHS to NUPE. NALGO has no direct political affiliations and its work on equal rights, part-time workers, and the defence of the public sector has a high profile. Both unions have positive policies with respect to public health care provision and lesbian and gay rights.

NUPE have published a well-circulated leaflet on 'AIDS Hysteria'. First produced in response to the public reaction to the death of the prison chaplain, it explains clearly and simply what AIDS is, how it is caught and who is at risk. Its Union journal has carried articles on AIDS on three occasions, and one letter. In September 1985, the Union published a report on AIDS from their Nurses' Group at St Mary's Hospital which identified the threat to service provision posed by government inaction.[9] The report dealt with the health and safety aspects of HIV infection in a positive and non-sensationalist way and gave detailed evidence of the effects of health service cutbacks on patient care. This was quickly followed up a month later by a second report which dealt specifically with the need for increased health service resources. The paper was a model of clarity, but received little publicity at the time. NUPE has also written to the Health Minister demanding a comprehensive health education programme, and more recently to all MPs demanding that resources be made available for a coordinated response to AIDS. In addition, a series of circulars have been sent to branches giving guidance on health and safety, and the Union's 1985 conference passed a resolution condemning the use of the infectious diseases regulations against people with AIDS. A detailed pamphlet on AIDS as an issue for NUPE and the Terrence Higgins Trust's leaflet 'Women and AIDS' have both been circulated to branches. At present NUPE is developing guidelines on good practice for shop stewards on how to handle HIV/AIDS cases. In terms of both quality and quantity, NUPE has maintained a consistent and positive approach to AIDS which has concentrated on putting the responsibility for action firmly in the hands of central government, whilst at the same time keeping its membership informed.

NALGO first issued advice to its branches around the same time as NUPE. This advice took the form of a briefing summarizing the contents of the ACDP guidelines with a commentary on them as well as information about HIV transmission. The Union has also distributed the Health Education Council's pamphlet 'Some facts about AIDS'. Early in 1985, when the panic surrounding AIDS was at its peak, NALGO produced a leaflet called 'AIDS — setting the record straight'. This leaflet concentrated on fighting homophobia, and stressed that prejudice was more dangerous than the disease. The first print run of this leaflet was exhausted within three weeks and in all 258,000 copies have been ordered by NALGO branches. The leaflet has been reproduced in the weekly newsletter to activists, and summarized in the Union journal. All 3000 branch equal opportunities officers and health and safety officers have also been issued with copies of the 'AIDS — a trade union issue' organizing pack, the Department of Employment pamphlet 'AIDS and employment' and the Terrence Higgins Trusts's leaflet 'Women and AIDS'.

A detailed policy document on the implications of AIDS for NALGO members was approved by the National Executive in mid-1985 and circulated to branches with advice on negotiating possible agreements to protect members who had AIDS or AIDS-related illnesses. The paper has been reproduced in full in the activists' newsletter, and in the Union's Research magazine. As a result of that paper, all NALGO's committees have been asked to ensure that service conditions claims are lodged with all national negotiating bodies to ensure that no members are discriminated against.

NALGO's 1986 annual conference adopted a detailed motion which outlined an overall strategy for dealing with the issues raised by AIDS, and took existing union policy one step further. In addition, NALGO organized a fringe meeting at the 1985 Trades Union Congress conference on behalf of the Terrence Higgins Trust, proposed motions on AIDS to the last two annual general meetings of the National Council for Civil Liberties and circulated an appeal for funds for Gay Sweatshop to allow them to stage the play *Compromised Immunity.*

Here then we have two trade unions, both prepared to tackle the issues raised by HIV and AIDS, but which have gone about this in very different ways. NUPE has put most of its emphasis on demanding action from central government. That has been the message which comes across clearly in most of its material. Next has been its concern for health and safety issues and finally it has addressed itself to discrimination. NALGO, on the other hand, has seen AIDS first as a threat to equal opportunities, second as a health and safety matter, and third as a conditions of service issue.

These differences of approach, however, are not simply subtle variations in emphases. The policies developed by these two unions emerged from the differing situations they found themselves in, and the different pressures they faced. NUPE is commonly seen as having a particularly high profile of fighting cuts in public sector service provision, and a large part of its resources over the past ten years have been diverted to that end. NUPE's members have borne the brunt of cuts and privatization far more than those of most other unions. Much of the pressure for action therefore came from branch activists such as the St Mary's Nurses Group who were already campaigning around the issue of resources, and who could clearly see the threat to patient care that central government inaction on AIDS posed. Second, many of its members were in day-to-day contact with the threat (real or imagined) of infection, and were demanding protection or reassurance. It was the pressure from these sources that helped shape NUPE's response. Although NUPE has a good policy on lesbian and gay rights, and has had so for many years, there is no organized focus for this activity within the Union.

NALGO, on the other hand, not only has a long and consistent policy of opposing heterosexism in the workplace, it also has a relatively good record of putting these policies into practice at local level. Many NALGO branches have campaigned on lesbian and gay rights, and in one case even took industrial action in support of a member victimized for being gay. [10] In addition NALGO has negotiated employment protection policies for lesbians and gay men in two of the industries it covers, and has attempted to do so in most others. More importantly, it has encouraged minority groups to organize separately within the union, and has by far the strongest and most active lesbian and gay group of any Union. Not surprisingly therefore, it was from this group of members, who found themselves increasingly under threat in the workplace, that the demand for action first came. The action they demanded was, in the first instance, a campaign aimed at educating and informing the members, and secondly, that the union negotiate protection from employers. With respect to health and safety issues relating to HIV infection, although NALGO issued sound advice very quickly, its members, being white-collar, were less likely to be directly involved with patient care. In consequence, the Union has not come under the same degree of pressure in this latter respect from its members as many other unions have done.

Planning for the Future

So far I have tried to show how the British trade union response to HIV infection and AIDS has not taken the form of a deliberate thought-out strategy coordinated by the union leadership. It has instead been reactive in nature, arising in response to grass roots pressures, not all of which have been for action of a positive nature. A number of unions, for example, have seen anti-gay motions come up from branches under the guise of concern and fear about AIDS.

The experience of NUPE and NALGO in this respect has been broadly mirrored by that of other unions. By and large, individual unions have reacted to specific cases and to specific pressures from members or groups of members. Many union head offices have little knowledge of HIV infection and AIDS and some have structures which make it hard for members to make their voice heard. In a large number of unions, equal opportunities issues around sexuality have yet to be taken up, and a few unions have a leadership which is itself openly and unashamedly homophobic in the stance it takes. [11]

However, it is not sufficient for trade unions to wait for pressure from their members before taking action on AIDS. The trade union movement needs to act proactively by developing a coordinated strategy for dealing positively with the complex issues raised by AIDS, rather than relying on 'knee-jerk' principles. It is clear that a more comprehensive approach is required. In planning this, problems arise from the fact that the membership of each union is different. Moreover, the outlook and general approach of individual unions covers a very wide spectrum indeed. There is no one strategy which could ideally cater for the needs of groups as diverse as the Health Visitors' Association and the National Union of Seamen. Each union must therefore develop a strategy that is geared towards meeting the needs of members and its own internal structure.

Nevertheless, it is possible, and I believe imperative, for the TUC to issue a basic framework containing guidance on those areas where there is a need for individual unions to develop policy. This should be done not with the intention that individual trade unions should just take these guidelines and adopt them, but with the view that they should be developed to suit the specific needs of their membership.

The basis for such a strategy already exists. The 'AIDS is a trade union issue' group have already distributed 6,500 copies of a comprehensive organizing pack for Trade Unions. [12] Sadly, however, the unions most using the pack are by and large those which have already done most.

What then are the main features of this coordinated strategy that trade unionists should be trying to develop? First, all unions need to adopt policies aimed at combatting discrimination against lesbians and gay men, publicize these amongst their membership, encourage lesbians and gay men to organize within the union, and seek agreements with employers that lesbians and gay men will not be discriminated against. Equally unions must be prepared to take up issues of racism in the workplace.

Second, there is a need for clear simple information about what AIDS is, what it is not, and how it is spread. Trade Unions should produce clear guidelines identifying the health and safety implications of HIV infection for their membership. Where appropriate, unions should demand that employers provide proper training, information and advice on the health and safety issues relating to HIV infection and AIDS, and ensure that any precautions necessary to protect workers are adequately financed and adhered to.

Next, unions should ensure that none of their members are dismissed or suspended because they have AIDS or HIV infection. No person should be redeployed unless at their own request, and any information on a person's health status must be confidential. Unions should resist any attempt to introduce compulsory HIV antibody testing, and should negotiate time-off agreements for people with AIDS or HIV infection, and for those who care for them.

The TUC, as well as individual trade unions, should campaign for adequate resources from central government for a comprehensive package to meet the challenge of AIDS. This means demanding the funding necessary to meet the cost of the National Health Service's AIDS-related caseload, a coordinated research programme, and a comprehensive and frank programme of health education. It means fighting for increased resources for local authorities to allow them to set up AIDS counselling and support groups. It also means calling on central government to provide greater funding for organizations like the Terrence Higgins Trust, the Haemophilia Society, Body Positive, local lesbian and gay switchboards and AIDS support groups. The fight against privatization within the National Health Service needs intensifying. In addition, central government should be asked to mount a campaign aimed at encouraging lesbians to donate blood, and to ensure that the Blood Transfusion Service is provided with sufficient resources to meet the extra burden HIV infection and AIDS has placed on it.

Finally, both the TUC and individual trade unions should campaign for the repeal of the Public Health (Infectious Diseases) Regulations 1985, which allow people with AIDS to be detained in hospital against their will, and resist any further attacks on civil liberties such as proposals to test those entering the country from black Africa.

Recommendations like these are not intended as a shopping list. They constitute a comprehensive and coherent strategy. The TUC may often be thought of as a great lumbering carthorse, but it does have the power, even under the present government, to help change public opinion and policy. But it is not enough to sit back demanding that the trade union leadership gets its act together. The impetus for action must come from below, for it is at this level that the policies will have to be implemented. A great deal of the work which some local authorities are now undertaking in terms of support and counselling has come about through pressure from local NALGO branches. Groups of local health workers have been instrumental in getting local health authorities to act on AIDS much more quickly than they otherwise would have.

Although this chapter has concentrated almost exclusively on what the trade union bureaucracy has or has not done, it is in the workplace that issues related to AIDS are, in the last analysis, tackled. The bureaucracy is important, because it has a vital role in formulating policy and disseminating information and it has been these processes that have been most focussed on in this chapter, but it is in local trade union branches that the real work will be done. To a large extent the impetus for this is likely to come from activists, many of whom are gay, and who are already under immense pressure as a result of the effect which AIDS has had on their own lives. Many others who are becoming active around the issue of AIDS have no previous experience of working within the often cumbersome trade union structures, and that is why material like the 'AIDS — A trade union issue' organizing pack is particularly useful.

It is now almost two years since the panic surrounding AIDS reached its peak, and the trade union movement is still groping around in the dark. Yet throughout that two years the government has continued to cut back National Health Service provision, lesbians and gay men have continued to be persecuted or ostracized at work, and people have continued to become infected because the government has refused to mount an explicit and hard hitting public health information programme.

There have of course been other issues for the trade union movement to give its attention to. Issues like mass unemployment, anti-union legislation, low pay, the miners' strike and privatization. But it is not an either/or situation. They are not faced with the option of either fighting privatization or developing a strategy on AIDS. It is not a choice of either fighting low pay or informing members about AIDS. They are part of the same fight — the fight for a fairer, more equal Britain, where health care, education, and the right to work are all given their proper status; where women, blacks, and lesbians and gays are given equal access to jobs and services, and where public services are seen as a public asset.

The government's failure to provide proper funding to deal with AIDS cannot be divorced from its policies concerning privatization and reducing public expenditure on the National Health Service. Nor can the right to job security for people with AIDS and lesbians and gays be seen in a separate context from demands for the right to work for all. The failure of the Conservative government to provide effective health education on AIDS, free from moralistic restraints, cannot be separated from its overall disastrous policies on both sex education and education in general. Over the next few years it is to be hoped that the British trade unions will learn that AIDS is far from an irrelevant issue in the fight against Thatcherism, and that people more generally will learn that trade unions are not peripheral to the fight against AIDS.

Notes

1 See for example the booklet *AIDS and Employment* published jointly in 1986 by the Department of Employment and the Health and Safety Executive.
2 See *AIDS — A Trade Union Issue.*
3 See report in *Capital Gay*, 8 November 1985.
4 See *Danger! Heterosexism at work*, London, GLC, 1986.
5 See *NCU Journal*, March 1985.
6 See *NATFHE Journal*, December 1985.
7 See the *New Statesman*, 7 November 1985 for a discussion of these issues.
8 See *Labour Research*, February 1986.
9 See *The AIDS Epidemic — A Time for Action*, London, NUPE.
10 Strike by Tower Hamlets NALGO, 1975.
11 See, *What About the Gay Workers?*, London, CHE.
12 Available from A-TUI, 15 Highstone, 84 Camden Rd, London NW1 9DY.

9
Health Education, HIV Infection and AIDS

Hilary Homans and Peter Aggleton

Many of the chapters in this book examine the social construction of AIDS as well as the ways in which HIV infection and its consequences have been misreported and misunderstood by lay people and professionals alike. The purpose of this chapter is to examine why a variety of health conditions which are to a large extent preventable continue to be transmitted at a worrying rate. In order to do this, we will document the philosophies that lie behind the actions of health educators working in the area of HIV infection and draw out the usefulness and limitations of the various styles or models of health education with which they work. Our analysis will focus on health education practice in Britain and elsewhere.

Before we can start to talk about the underlying philosophy and efficacy of different models of health education, we need to be clear what it is what we are educating people about. Because of this we need to start by being clear what health itself is. There is considerable disagreement among lay people and health professionals (be they health educators, physicians, medical sociologists or practitioners of complementary medicine) about the nature of health, and in consequence there are a variety of lay and professional definitions of health. Conventionally, distinctions are often made between *bio-medical* definitions of health as the absence of disease, *social* definitions of health as the absence of illness and *holistic* definitions of health as a positive ideal encompassing (amongst other things) physical, mental, social, spiritual and sexual well-being. In the discussions they have about health and in the interventions that follow from these, lay people and health professionals use these definitions variably — switching paradigms as the occasion requires.

Within the context of HIV infection and AIDS, these different definitions become all the more significant because to a greater or lesser extent they inform the different lay and professional understandings of HIV infection and AIDS that abound. In our earlier work we have examined a variety of different lay and professional beliefs about HIV infection and AIDS (Aggleton and Homans, 1987; Aggleton, Homans and Warwick, 1987). With respect to professional explanations, a clear distinction can be drawn between those theories that were popular amongst physicians and scientists in the early 1980s before HIV was isolated and identified, and the theories that have come to be widely accepted within these same communities since then. Professional explanations popular in the early 1980s included immune overload theory (Johnson and Ho, 1985; Liscombe, 1985), single agent microbial theory (Auerbach *et al*, 1984; Gazzard *et al*, 1984) and multifactorial theory (Sonnabend *et al*, 1983; Adkins, 1985). After the identification of HIV in 1984, different kinds of professional explanation began to gain acceptance. These included the view that (i) HIV is a necessary and sufficient cause of AIDS (Gallo *et al*, 1985); (ii) HIV is a necessary but not sufficient cause of AIDS (Pinching, 1986; Weber *et al*, 1986); and (iii) AIDS is an opportunistic marker of infection by an as yet unidentified agent (Ortleb, 1985a-c: 1986a-f). All these professional explanations have been put forward to explain the same phenomenon and their existence poses something of a challenge for those who want to fully understand the current state of play with respect to mainstream medical and scientific understandings of AIDS.

Concurrent with professional explanations such as these are lay theories about the nature and origins of AIDS. In our research amongst young people (reported elsewhere in this book) we have identified four different kinds of lay theory of causation amongst the young people we have interviewed. These lay theories emphasize endogenous factors, exogenous variables, personal (ir)responsibility and supernatural intervention respectively. We (and others) have also begun to chart some of the ways in which HIV infection and AIDS are popularly understood. Of particular importance within this context are some of the ambiguities and confusions that stem from the popular conceptions of AIDS as a 'disease' and of there being an 'AIDS virus' that causes it. In reality of course AIDS (Acquired Immune Deficiency Syndrome) is as its name suggests a *syndrome* not a disease. As such, it is a medically defined condition which requires a person to be first infected with the virus HIV, and then to develop other opportunistic infections or diseases. This combination of events (not infection by HIV alone) constitutes the syndrome that is referred to as AIDS. People cannot therefore 'catch' AIDS, the syndrome is not contagious and is in no way transmissible from one person to another. What may be transmitted between two people is a virus (HIV), and this as we know only takes place via 'critical quantities' and 'critical routes'. To some, these distinctions may appear a matter of semantics, but to those with HIV infection and to the people who care for them, they are crucial issues.

In this chapter we will therefore critically review some of the different approaches that can be taken within the context of education about HIV infection and AIDS. We will focus attention particularly on the strategies that can be used to help groups clarify what they already know about the issues involved as well as identify the steps that need to be taken to make this information available to others. Our discussion of these issues will be illustrated by examples taken from contemporary health education practice in Britain and elsewhere.

Health Education and Health Promotion

There are at least two significant dimensions to health education today. On the one hand it is likely to involve learning about diseases, the effects that they have on our health, how to avoid them and how, if we become diseased, health can be restored. On the other hand, health education can also include developing a more sophisticated appreciation of the social factors affecting our health, learning about our sensuality and our sexuality and acquiring insight into the ways in which different states of health and well-being are socially constructed.

Some of these latter aspects of health education are also referred to as *health promotion*. In January 1984, the World Health Organization launched a new programme of health promotion with five key principles (WHO, 1984). These identify some of the key components within health promotion.

> ... Health promotion involves the population as a whole in the context of their everyday life, rather than focussing on people at risk for specific diseases ... is directed towards action on the determinants or causes of health ... combines diverse, but complementary, methods or approaches ... aims particularly at effective and concrete public participation ... health professionals — particularly in primary health care — have an important role in nurturing and enabling health promotion ...

This definition of health promotion is particularly pertinent to our analysis for two reasons. First, it operates with a broader definition of health education than is the case with some more 'traditional' notions about the role of the health educator. Second, while it recognizes that there can be many ways of promoting health, it places particular emphasis on participatory forms of learning about and involvement in health issues.

The history of health education indicates how participation in the processes of health has not always been an ideal towards which health educators have worked. Lussier (1984) for example has described how health education originally emerged from the distinct disciplines of education and medicine in the nineteenth century as a set of pedagogic practices associated with sanitary reform and hygiene education. Early styles of health education were largely didactic in their emphasis, and aimed mainly to provide information about disease transmission and containment.

Changes in patterns of morbidity and mortality, as well as a growing recognition that personal lifestyles were implicated in the causation of ill-health, subsequently shifted the emphasis within health education from disease processes to personal behaviour. Nevertheless, the emphasis still lay on information giving with the intention of bringing about changes in personal lifestyles and habits. This more modern approach to health education has been criticized for being too negative in its tone — Don't drink! Don't smoke! Get plenty of exercise!' — and for being too individualistic in its orientation (Naidoo, 1986; Rodmell and Watt, 1986). By way of contrast, some of the most recent initiatives in health education have focussed on health enhancement, and a growing number of health educators argue that the impact of social, environmental and economic factors affecting health needs to be more closely examined (Draper *et al*, 1980; Mitchell, 1982; Moran, 1986; Cribb, 1986).

These various ideas about health education can be related to our earlier discussion of the different ways in which health is understood. Thus, disease oriented biomedical understandings of health frequently inform preventive approaches in health education which emphasize the importance of changes in individual behaviour. More social concepts of health which acknowledge the role played by existing social relations in structuring health inequalities often suggest health education strategies concerned with community development and social change. Holistic concepts of health, on the other hand, are likely to connect with styles of health education which are more self-empowering in their emphasis.

Models of Health Education

In recent years there has been a great deal of debate about the different paradigms or *models of health education* within which health educators can operate. Unfortunately, much of this discussion has confused, rather than clarified, the central issues as we perceive them. A brief review of the main themes within this debate would seem useful before we attempt to identify the strengths and limitations of some of the strategies currently being used in AIDS education.

One of the major problems in existing debates about models of health education is the failure to clearly distinguish between the *content* of health education intervention, the different *goals* of health education initiatives and the *means* by which these might be achieved. A clear analysis of models of health education needs to distinguish systematically between the means and outcomes of health education interventions. Such an analysis has recently been put forward by French and Adams (1986) who have identified three broad paradigms within which health education can take place. They call these the behaviour change paradigm, the self-empowerment paradigm and the collective action paradigm. The goals of each of these approaches are as follows. The behaviour change model seeks to 'improve health by changing people's behaviour', the self-empowerment model attempts to 'improve health by developing people's ability to understand and control their health status to whatever extent is possible within their environmental circumstances' and the collective action model is concerned to 'improve health by changing environmental, social and economic factors through community involvement and action'.

In addition to specifying the goals of different kinds of health education, French and Adams also specify the means by which these might be achieved as well as the criteria by which successful intervention within each of these three paradigms might be evaluated. The clarity of the conceptual framework which they offer makes it particularly useful as a foundation for analyzing health education relating to HIV infection and AIDS. In order to do this we will take the first two models of health education identified by French and Adams — the behaviour change and the self-empowerment models — and we will add to these a third which is more community oriented and a fourth which is socially transformatory. While French and Adams argue that their collective action model will lead to social change, we feel that a more careful analysis is required of the limitations which often prevent community health initiatives from actually achieving social change. In this respect our analysis responds to the challenge posed by Watt (1986), Beattie (1986) and others who have been concerned to distinguish between different kinds of community-based health education.

The Behaviour Change Model

Earlier we referred to the connection between biomedical understandings of health and disease and health education which is concerned with changes in individual behaviour. We will now attempt to explore more fully the implications of this paradigm for effective education about AIDS.

Biomedical notions of health frequently emphasize the need for disease prevention and, in terms of learning about and coping with disease, it is sometimes useful to distinguish between three levels at which prevention can take place — the primary level, the secondary level and the tertiary level. Primary prevention focusses on the healthy population and aims to encourage health promoting behaviour. Secondary prevention on the other hand is more concerned with the early detection and treatment of disease and with the provision of information on how health can be restored. Tertiary prevention is aimed more directly at people who are chronically or terminally ill and is particularly concerned with maximizing their remaining potential for living.

In general terms, biomedical understandings of health and disease have encouraged preventive forms of health education in which priority is given to the provision of information and the promotion of screening services. The usual aim of these interventions is to bring about changes in behaviour so that individuals can lead healthier lives.

Within the context of AIDS education, many central government initiatives as well as those taking place within health districts and local authorities have their origins in this model of health education. Much of the discussion about AIDS education in Britain and America has focussed on the ways in which people can be encouraged to change their behaviour so that they do not put themselves at risk of infection. In some literature, lifestyles (being gay, being 'promiscuous', being an injecting drug user, being a prostitute etc) are seen as the factors which put people at risk. Efforts should therefore be made to encourage them to change their behaviour. A mass media approach is often recommended as the most appropriate means by which these changes can be brought about. This might aim to provide information to increase knowledge and hopefully produce changes in both attitudes and behaviour. Leaflets, posters, television and newspaper advertisements are the main methods likely to be used to bring about this kind of behaviour change. This is most clearly the approach adopted in the campaign launched in Britain by the Department of Health in the spring 1986 and in early 1987.

However, past evaluations of mass media campaigns such as these tend to show that the increase in knowledge that they produce is likely to be short-lived and that the shifts in attitudes they create are likely to be slight. Indeed, as Gatherer *et al* (1979) have observed, sometimes there may even be 'shifts in attitude in the opposite direction to that desired'.

In relation to the 1986 Department of Health campaign, there was criticism of the strategies used right from the start. *The Guardian* (1986) claimed that the resources made available for the initial stages of such an important campaign (about £2.5 million) were insufficient for the task in hand. Others were more critical of the methods that the campaign employed. Adler (1986), for example, saw newspaper advertisements on their own as having limited value, and argued instead for a comprehensive campaign involving television, radio and leaflets to every household. This in fact followed at the end of the year. Other commentators expressed concern about the content of the campaign, making particular reference to the language used (Mills *et al*, 1986), the information given about the virus and the fact that the campaign's messages seemed to be addressed largely at gay men rather than the population at large (BMJ, 1986; Wells, 1986).

Subsequent evaluation of the effectiveness of the first stages of this campaign has not been particularly encouraging. Market research carried out for the Department of Health immediately after the campaign suggested that only about a quarter of a sample of 1400 adults aged between 18–64 years were aware of the advertising involved (DHSS, 1986). An independent postal survey conducted in Southampton revealed that only 31 per cent of respondents were aware of the advertisements (Mills *et al*, 1986), and concluded somewhat pessimistically that the campaign,

> ... seems to have had little effect on the public's knowledge of AIDS (and) the increased publicity may have caused some confusion about the principal causes of AIDS ... (cited in Wells, 1986)

At the time of writing, the 1987 Department of Health campaign, which involved the distribution of the leaflet 'AIDS: Don't die of ignorance' to every household in Britain plus television, radio, poster and newspaper advertising is still in progress, and evaluation of its effectiveness is only just beginning to appear. However, discussions in recent training sessions we have facilitated as part of our work on the *Learning About AIDS* project indicate that one of the unintended consequences of the recent campaign has been to suggest that everyone is at risk of AIDS, whether or not they involve themselves in activities which are risky within the context of HIV infection. This has tended to confuse people and raise anxiety rather than inform and reassure.

The most effective interventions within the behaviour change model of health education tend to be those where the behaviour change required is a single action. Evaluation also seems to show that the most effective way of spreading information appears to be through word of mouth and personal contact, not through the mass media (Gatherer *et al*, 1979). This latter point is particularly relevant to any discussion of AIDS education, especially when we take into account the existence of lay beliefs about health and illness in general and about HIV infection and AIDS in particular. Any campaign which focusses solely on biomedical aspects of the disease at the expense of lay beliefs and that uses impersonal media messages rather than personal networks is likely to be severely limited in its overall effectiveness (WHO, 1986).

There is now a growing body of literature which suggests that within the context of AIDS education, the provision of information on its own does not appear to be effective. Recent research in the United States for example has shown that even in areas where there is a high incidence of HIV infection and where there have been sustained public information campaigns, knowledge about AIDS among school children is no better than in areas which do not share these characteristics (DiClemente *et al*, 1986). Yet individuals who are themselves part of a community perceived to be 'at risk' have changed their sexual behaviour quite dramatically. Silverman (1986) for example has reported a 75 per cent decrease in the incidence of rectal gonorrhoea amongst gay men between 1980 and 1984 and contrasts these findings with those for weight reduction programmes where there has typically been only a 5 per cent decrease in weight over the same time period. Studies by McKusick *et al* (1985) also show the there have been dramatic changes in behaviour amongst gay men living on the West Coast of America. In the light of this evidence it would seem that motivation to protect oneself and others from disease may be more pronounced among gay men than among the population as a whole in relation to general health issues. In areas of America where the incidence of HIV infection is low, Shaw and Palco (1986) argue that safer sexual practices are not taken so seriously. They suggest that in these instances the lower risk population should be given education in decision making and risk evaluation. In this respect much can be learned from one of the first AIDS education campaigns devised by the Los Angeles Cooperative Risk Reduction Service. This too was developed within the framework of the behaviour change model of health education and sought to enhance awareness and provide education about alternative forms of low risk sexual behaviour. Using the theme 'LA cares ... like a mother', the campaign utilized posters, public service announcements, display advertisements and handout material (including calling cards and pamphlets) to communicate a number of simple health education messages linked to discrete and specific behavioural changes. These messages included 'Say "no" to unsafe sex', 'Don't forget your rubbers' and 'Don't use needles'. One of the most striking aspects of the campaign was its use of a positive figure — 'mother' — who appeared on all the publicity material associated with the project (as well as at live appearances) giving sound advice to her various 'sons' on what they should and should not do. 'Mother' was portrayed by the distinctive actress Zelda Rubinstein, and her 'sons' were deliberately chosen so as to project, in the words of the advertising agency handling the campaign, 'a slight sexuality as an attention getting device'.

In distinction to the Department of Health's campaigns here in Britain, the LA cares initiative sought to personalize its messages. As part of this strategy, 'mother' attended small group meetings around the city of Los Angeles and organized parties and meetings at which she urged others to spread her health education messages on a one-to-one basis. While the campaign was originally devised to meet the health education needs of Los Angeles' gay community, there is no reason to believe that similar approaches may not be effective among other client groups.

Some British health education initiatives within the behaviour change paradigm have tried to operate on a one to one basis. According to Gatherer *et al* (1979), the overall success of these varies from between 10–36 per cent. In relation to AIDS education, most of these interventions have so far taken place within the context of pre-test and post-test counselling and there have been reports that interventions of this kind can be relatively effective in bringing about enduring changes in behaviour (Green, 1986a and 1986b). It is only fair to point out, however, that the amount of counselling provision available is as yet limited and many opportunities for counselling before and after HIV antibody testing are not fully utilized because of demands on the service, lack of time and a shortage of trained counsellors. In consequence, some 'counselling' sessions may turn out to be little more than rather impersonal information-giving exercises rather than counselling in a more growth oriented or therapeutic sense.

No matter what approach they adopt, behaviour change models of health education lay themselves open to the criticism that they focus too much on the role of the 'expert' whose task it is to 'tell' the client 'what to do'. To be on the receiving end of a health education intervention of this kind may be a profoundly disempowering experience for many people. An example of this is provided by a recent critique of the Gay Men's Health Crisis '800 Men Project' in America — a project which focussed on behaviour change and the control and management of individual sexual practices. In his evaluation of this programme, Silin (1987) argues,

> Programs such as the 800 Project are built on the belief that we can change our behaviour while ignoring questions of the deeper meanings with which these may be charged by different elements of society ... ironically, we appear (by doing this) to be participating in the re-medicalization of homosexuality, a process that began in the nineteenth century with the coming of the word 'homosexual'.

Recent developments in community medicine and community health, as well as academic debate within the spheres of sociology, philosophy, psychology and health education has led to an enhanced consumer awareness of the benefits to be gained from direct involvement in health-related issues. In consequence, there is a growing advocacy for styles of health education which operate with a commitment to notions of self-empowerment. We will examine these in detail in the next section.

The Self Empowerment Model

Organizations such as the Terrence Higgins Trust, the Haemophilia Society, the Royal College of Nursing, the Confederation of Health Service Employees, the National Association of Local Government Officers, the National Union of Public Employees and the National Union of Students have produced a wide range of information about HIV infection and AIDS, recognizing that in the first instance this material can only increase people's knowledge about the disease and that, on its own, it is unlikely to lead to enduring changes in behaviour. Some of these organizations are also acutely conscious of the need for this information to be located within the context of people's everyday lives and encountered in a form which permits fears and anxieties to be discussed and allayed where possible. This process can be facilitated using a self-empowerment model of health education which encourages the use of participatory learning.

Self-empowerment is a term which is frequently used in health education but rarely defined. We use the term to describe the process by which people develop skills, understandings and awareness so that they can act on the basis of rational choice rather than irrational feelings (Satow, 1987). A self-empowerment model of health education is therefore one in which the individual uses her or his personal resources to the full, thereby maximizing their chances of leading a healthy life. Tatchell (1986) and Spence (1986) present detailed accounts of different self-empowerment strategies that are used within the context of HIV infection and AIDS. In particular, they seek to demonstrate, from rather different standpoints, how people diagnosed as HIV antibody positive or as having AIDS can 'reclaim their power' and thereby 'survive'.

Self-empowerment techniques have often been promoted in books and training materials concerned with assertiveness (Dickson, 1982), sexuality and personal relationships (Human Rights Foundation, 1984; Clarity Collective, 1985; Dickson, 1985; Dixon, 1986; Szirom and Dyson, 1986) and are all based on methods of learning which are participative in character. This form of learning is advocated as being more successful because the learner is actively encouraged to participate in the learning programme, to explore their own values and beliefs, and to develop an understanding of the extent to which factors such as past socialization and position in society affect the choices that each of us make.

The concept of self-empowerment is, however, problematic, and this is in part related to the concept of power with which it operates. Some analysts define power in constant-sum terms (either you have it or you don't), others such as Parsons (1957) define power more expansively as a resource, a facility, a capacity or an ability. It is with this latter use that proponents of self-empowerment feel most comfortable. They see power as a resource shared by all individuals, but as something which is in some people undeveloped. According to this perspective, the process of self-empowerment and the skills that are thereby developed are sufficient for the individual to actually become more powerful.

The major problem with this approach, of course, is that it marginalizes the effects that systematically structured inequalities have in limiting the expression of power. Gender, class, race and age (amongst other variables) all set limits on the autonomy of individuals and groups, and it is arguable whether self-empowerment alone is sufficient to effectively resist the constraints imposed by social structures such as these. Someone who has been through an assertion training course or rebirthing, for example, may *feel* more powerful, more self-important and more confident after the experience, but unless the conditions which led to their original feeling of worthlessness and powerlessness are changed, these enhanced feelings may evaporate on the next occasion that their cause is encountered.

It is not enough for individuals to participate in their own learning experiences. They also need to be involved in the decision-making processes that affect their day to day lives. Self-empowerment can be a first stage in enabling people to gain confidence, wider participation in social issues would seem essential if the ultimate origins of ill-health are to be tackled.

The Community Oriented Model

Community oriented models of health education attempt to move away from the notion that the individual is responsible for his or her own health to suggest that people should collectively identify and act upon the environmental and community-based factors that affect their health. The term 'community' is however also problematic as Watt (1986) has recently shown in her analysis of these styles of health education which have community intervention as their focus. It is often used loosely to indicate a shared environment identified by certain characteristics — for example the 'gay community', the 'black community', 'working class' communities. This particular usage tends to conjure up images of homogeneous groups of people working and living in similar environments. But such imagery can be very misleading since it obscures the differences that exist within each of these groups — a view which is often reinforced by media representations of these same groups. For example, recent media reporting on gay lifestyles has tended to imply that all (or the majority) of gay men have multiple sexual partners. Nothing could be further from the truth, and on an age-for-age basis there may well exist the same diversity of relationships among gay men as can be found among their heterosexual counterparts.

See Mike Kelly's article on health promotion

Bearing these difficulties of terminology and meaning in mind, it is possible to identify two ways in which intervention has taken place within a community oriented approach to health education. We can call these top-down and grass-roots initiatives (Beattie, 1986). Generally speaking the former kind of intervention focusses on issues which health educators themselves define as important. The impact of initiatives which have this kind of emphasis is often limited by the extent to which the priorities of health educators coincide with those of their client groups and with those of health and social services administrators.

Grass-roots initiatives on the other usually arise from the concerns of community groups organized around particular health issues. Some of these groups may be completely autonomous of the medical profession and the health service, whereas others may rely for their success on medical patronage. The overall effectiveness of these groups lies in their being able to identify their own health-related needs and plan programmes to meet these. The limitations they face are often financial.

In relation to HIV infection and AIDS, the Terrence Higgins Trust provides a useful illustration of a self-help group founded by gay men to provide information, education and counselling support for other gay men. Its trustees include physicians and representatives from other professional and lay organizations. Since it was originally founded, however, the scope of its activities has been extended dramatically to include service provision for other groups including injecting drug users, women and church-goers. The Terrence Higgins Trust's lack of financial support has often been commented on, and the expansion of its activities into spheres of practice very different from those which it was originally intended to serve has not been without its costs. In recent months, these affected both those working within it, be they paid or voluntary workers, and those seeking to use its services.

The work of the Terrence Higgins Trust and Body Positive (a self-help group providing support for those who are diagnosed as HIV antibody positive) in Britain is very similar to that of similar organizations in the United States. In the latter context, the success of self-help groups like these in providing realistic and appropriate information on safer sex and health education has been widely recognized as a significant factor both in slowing down the rate of transmission of HIV amongst gay men and in promoting health more generally.

In Britain we currently do not have national data about the adoption of safer forms of sexual practice, although Coxon's work at University College, Cardiff (reported on elsewhere in this book) may in time provide this. However, there have been recent falls nationally in the incidence of acute gonorrhoea among gay men attending clinics for the treatment of sexually transmitted diseases (CDR, 1986). These national figures are closely paralled by local reports from those areas of the country where HIV infection is believed to be most widespread (Gellan and Ison, 1986). Statistics relating to a declining incidence of gonorrhoea are currently taken by some as a useful indicator of the extent to which safer forms of sexual expression are being practised. A survey carried out by Burton *et al* (1986) showed that 95 per cent of 300 gay men interviewed said they had received some information about safer sex from within the gay community and that 75 per cent of the same were following the guidelines.

These findings suggest that community-focussed health education can be successful in reducing the transmission of HIV infection among gay men at least, and the apparent success of strategies such as these reflects the appropriateness both of the health education messages with which they operate and the methods used to get these across. This is in sharp contrast to the behaviour change approach to AIDS education which we referred to earlier. There is a tremendous difference between groups of people being responsible for their own learning and situations in which 'sex experts' or health professionals attempt to change the behaviour of others.

As part of this community oriented approach, gay pubs and clubs have frequently been used as venues for meetings and for the dissemination of information on a one to one or small group basis. Moreover, a number of community oriented interventions have aimed not only to persuade gay men to adopt safer sexual practices but to provide health education more generally. Both Body Positive and the Terrence Higgins Trust stress the value of conventional health education messages about cigarette smoking, alcohol consumption, balanced nutrition, exercise and adequate sleep.

In the United States, and to a lesser but growing extent in Britain, community-oriented programmes such as these have been taken one step further through the setting up of extensive support systems involving crisis intervention workers and 'buddies'. Whereas the task of the former may be to provide support and reassurance on occasions when there is particular distress, the latter provide support for People with AIDS on a more enduring basis and may mediate between their clients and health care professionals. One particular initiative, the San Francisco based *Stop AIDS Project* believes that 'educational efforts should focus less on teaching the specifics of how to eroticize safer sex than on altering perceptions about community norms (and) establishing safer sex legitimacy' (Silin, 1987). This project is sub-titled 'a community experiment in communication' and is particularly concerned to be identified as a grass-roots, self-help initiative.

There is some evidence, therefore, that community-oriented approaches to AIDS education can be very successful in meeting a wide range of health-related needs. However, there is also a growing recognition that if AIDS education is to have long-term effectiveness, health educational interventions must be linked to changes in policy and legislation. As Silin (1987) says in relation to the *Stop AIDS Project*.

... While we can each play a role in ending the epidemic by practising safer sex, as a community we must also learn to fight for the funding, legal protections and attitudinal transformations necessary to ensure our future survival ...

Commitments like these can be seen as part of a more socially transformatory style of AIDS education.

The Socially Transformatory Model and AIDS Education

Recently a number of factors have given new impetus to the identification of forms of health education which are more embracing in their effects than those so far described. Some health educators have grown critical of the conservatism of traditional modes of professional practice operating with a commitment to behaviour change, self-empowerment or community action (Adams, 1985). These approaches, it is said, can do little to challenge the pervasive inequalities of power in society which affect the choices people make and limit opportunities for healthier forms of living. Other health educators have grown more acutely conscious of the health-related demands of divergent popular constituencies such as working class people, women, ethnic minority communities, the elderly, the disabled, lesbians and gay men (categories which are not, of course, used here exclusively).

As if to echo these sentiments, in a recent evaluation of AIDS training programmes in Britain, health education officers who participated in the study recognized that some problems to do with HIV infection and AIDS 'cannot be solved through training alone' (Craig, 1987). They identified lack of resources, staff and time as factors contributing to the difficulties they were encountering in planning appropriate AIDS education programmes.

In contrast to behaviour change, self-empowerment and community-oriented models of health education, socially transformatory paradigms have the potential to enhance individual health and well-being *and* to bring about far reaching social change throughout society. We can distinguish between four interrelated aspects of society which educators working with a commitment to social transformation will need to address — ideas, social relations, political processes and resource allocation.

Ideas

First, changes are likely to be necessary at the level of ideas. Much present medical knowledge about the causes of disease and ill health needs to be demystified and replaced by more accessible medical understandings in which scientific arguments are clearly separated from moral considerations. For example, present medical knowledge does not suggest that it is the number of partners *per se* which increases the likelihood of HIV infection. Rather, the particular acts that are engaged in with these partners are crucial in determining whether or not the virus is transmitted. Non-penetrative forms of sexual expression which do not involve the exchange of body fluids do not result in the transmission of the virus. Yet in our experience, few people seem aware of this, believing instead that medical evidence says that a high number of sexual partners will *by itself* increase the risk of infection.

In addition, attempts to encourage a reassessment of the nature of disability are required. As we mentioned earlier, people can have potentially fatal diseases and not be ill. We need also to remember that people with special physical and mental needs still have rights. At the level of ideas we are presented with a challenge to link the needs of those diagnosed as HIV antibody positive, or as having Persistent Generalized Lymphadenopathy, AIDS Related Complex or AIDS to specific rights, be these at the level of access to resources, service provision or interpersonal relations. Unless these connections are made, the full impact of receiving one of these diagnoses for the person concerned may continue to go unrecognized by the person making the diagnosis.

There is also a need to personalize and rehumanize the consequences of HIV infection so that those who are affected come once more to be seen as human beings with valuable qualities and important contributions to make to society.

Within the context of AIDS education, the connection between popular perceptions of the syndrome and notions of 'contagion' and 'plague' need to be critically explored. Patton's (1985) recent analysis of the relationship between germ theory and popular understandings of sexuality begins this task admirably. So long as people still believe that the virus can be 'caught' from being in the same room as a person with AIDS, there will be serious implications for the quality of care they deliver. A number of local authority initiatives are attempting to challenge these ideas through educational programmes for home care workers (NUPE Journal, 1987).

Finally, educators working with a socially transformatory ethic will need to address the fears and prejudices that underpin homophobic and anti-gay responses — be these within media representations of AIDS (including it is sad to say some health education resources being produced locally), the behaviour of particular health care workers or within the institutionalized practices of health and social service provision itself. As Richardson (1987) has recently put it, 'homophobia and anti-lesbianism, not AIDS, is the root of the problem'.

Social Relations

We have already begun to move beyond the realm of ideas alone to talk about changes in social relations. Undoubtedly some of the greatest challenges to be faced in the next few years by health educators committed to social transformation will be those concerned with fostering an increased understanding, compassion and concern for those who have (or who are assumed to have) HIV infection. Already criteria of moral worth have been established separating supposedly 'innocent' and 'guilty' victims of the disease. On a day to day basis, these criteria can be used as legitimating devices by which to deny interpersonal contact, but they may subsequently be used to restrict service provision to particular client groups. In the popular press, suggestions have already been made to visibly identify members of the 'at risk' groups who are seen as the 'guilty' transmitters of the disease. Health educators with a commitment to social justice can play a role locally in monitoring any differentiation of service provision along these grounds. Increasingly, they may feel the necessity to act 'politically' as the advocates and allies of certain client groups, especially in relation to challenging discrimination against people with AIDS.

Those who work within a socially transformatory model of health education will also find themselves considering the extent to which their work should be restricted solely to their professional sphere of practice. At least four arenas of intervention are open to health educators who desire to extend their role. *Personally*, changes in lifestyles and patterns of sexual behaviour may have to be made. Health educators for example may wish to explore safer sexual practices within the context of their own lifestyles. *Professionally*, contact can be fostered with organizations conventionally seen as beyond the remit of present health education practice. These may include gay and lesbian community groups, body positive groups, support groups for injecting drug users, prostitutes' collectives, and trade unions implementing programmes of AIDS education within the workplace. At a *peer group* level, it may be necessary to educate colleagues and friends who are less committed to initiatives which aim to achieve more than behaviour change or self-empowerment. Finally, for some health educators there is also an arena of *parental* intervention within the home and elsewhere.

At one level, the AIDS crisis provides opportunities for a radical re-orientation of sexual expression away from acts which are narrowly associated with bodily penetration and procreation. Health educators working to achieve these goals could form productive alliances with those already working in women's health (and elsewhere). Some women's groups are already advocating assertion training for women so that they will have more confidence in negotiating sexual encounters and in saying 'no' to risky sexual practices. Prostitutes also are becoming involved in training sessions demonstrating how to use condoms without their client's knowledge. Whilst these moves can be seen as part of a self-empowering process, they need to be understood within the context of the unequal power relationships between heterosexual men and women and the way in which sexual encounters are most usually organized around male sexual pleasure (Pollock, 1985). As Coward (1987) has recently commented, AIDS is going to create a 'sexual revolution' and it is important that women do not lose out:

> ... Men and women have different interests at stake in any possible sexual revolution and the crisis produced by AIDS may well have different implications for men and women ... women have been bearing the brunt of making sex safe for men in the past ... sexuality could be re-defined as something other than male discharge into any kind of receptacle ... In this new context where penetration might literally spell death, there's a chance for a massive re-learning about sexuality ...

Political Processes

Politically, health educators committed to social transformation are likely to work towards securing a more genuinely participatory politics of AIDS. At one level this may involve them providing opportunities and occasions when people most affected by AIDS can meet to identify and systematize their experiences and insights. As a result, people may become more critically conscious of the possibilities and limitations associated with existing health and social service provision. Health educators can also be involved in creating popular alliances between health care workers at different levels within the health service, the various community groups with an interest in HIV infection and AIDS, trades unions and others campaigning nationally for a restructuring of health and social service provision. These alliances could subsequently generate new ideas for health education intervention. Efforts could also be made to explore similarities and differences of approach within the context of trade union responses to AIDS (see Robertson's chapter in this book) as well as the appropriateness of various strategies in meeting local needs.

Resource Allocation

Finally, attention can usefully be given to a consideration of the resource implications associated with HIV infection and AIDS. Health educators committed to socially transformation have an important role to play in educating those who control access to resources such as housing, social, service and health care provision and insurance benefits. These issues are now of paramount importance if service provision is to be developed which is responsive to the needs of people with AIDS, those who are HIV antibody positive and those who are perceived as being in an 'at risk' group. Already in Britain steps are being taken in this direction by the Terrence Higgins Trust and the London Lighthouse Project.

Attention may also need to be focussed on the extent to which central government has (or has not) regarded it as a priority to fund basic medical research into vaccines, treatments and therapies related to AIDS as well as enquiry on the social and behavioural aspects of HIV infection. Local and central government politicians, civil servants and others with power to influence resource allocation could justifiably find themselves the targets of intervention within a socially transformatory paradigm. The Institute of Medicine (1987) in America has recently noted that whilst virologic research has received 'reasonable' levels of funding over the years, there has been 'chronic inadequate funding' of behavioural and social scientific enquiry. According to this report, the latter kind of research would not only enable the development of effective educational programmes, it could also,

> ... contribute to the development of informed public policies that reduce the public's fear of AIDS and discriminatory practices towards AIDS sufferers. And it can guide the establishment of improved health care and social services that further the ability to treat AIDS patients effectively, humanely and at reasonable cost ...

An example of the beginnings of a socially transformatory approach in Britain can be seen in the strategies recently adopted by Oxford City Council. According to Miller (1987), the city has tried to achieve five rather different sets of goals via its AIDS education initiatives. First, efforts have been made to locate work on AIDS and HIV infection firmly within the context of the city's other public health initiatives. Second, planning has taken place to try to ensure that the city's own services and those of other bodies are fully prepared for the implications of AIDS and HIV infection within the population of Oxford. Third, a series of positive health initiatives have been taken with the intention of preventing the spread of infection, dispelling panic and integrating AIDS and HIV into the health concerns of the community. Fourth, there have been efforts to maintain the equal opportunities policy of the City Council and to ensure that AIDS and HIV infection are not used to deny civil liberties. Finally, in planning this work the City Council has entered into collaboration with the local health authority, community organizations and others in order to maximize the effects of the strategy. It is too early to predict what the outcome of wide ranging interventions like this will be. Undoubtedly there will be struggles over the implementation of a wide ranging package of health education measures such as these and it is by no means certain that the outcome of initiatives within Oxford will be as planned.

Undoubtedly one of the challenges to which an integrated and radical programme of health education such as this will have to respond is that posed by creeping professionalization of practice. Health educators who see themselves as isolated radicals — as vanguards of a process of social transformation which will lead to a more equitable distribution of health-related life chances — may too easily find themselves removed from the grass roots concerns of those most affected by the AIDS crisis. Constant vigilance will be needed if socially transformatory styles of AIDS education are to be both meaningful and critical (Aggleton and Whitty, 1986).

Conclusions

In this chapter we have attempted to review some of the main features of four rather different kinds of AIDS education. In doing so we have tried to identify the strengths and weaknesses of a range of contemporary initiatives both in Britain and elsewhere. This kind of exercise, in which health educators stand back momentarily from their everyday work to critically evaluate the effects of the interventions they are involved with, is essential if we are to develop programmes of AIDS education which combine their desire for effectiveness with a respect for the dignity and true diversity of human experience.

References

ADAMS, L. (1985) 'Health education — In whose interest?', unpublished MA dissertation, University of London, Kings College.

ADKINS, B. (1985) 'Looking at AIDS in totality' — A conversation with Joseph Sonnabend, *New York Native*, 7 October, pp. 21–5.

ADLER, M. (1986) 'Time for honest talk on AIDS', *The Times*. 8 July.

AGGLETON, P. J. and HOMANS, H. (1987) *Educating about AIDS*, Bristol, National Health Service Training Authority.

AGGLETON, P. J., HOMANS, H. and WARWICK, I. (1987) 'Health education sexuality and AIDS', paper given at the Xth International Conference on the sociology of Education, Birmingham, January 1987, to appear in BARTON, L. and WALKER, S. (Eds.) *The Politics of Schooling*, Milton Keynes, Open University Press.

AGGLETON, P. J. and WHITTY, G. J. (1986) 'Components of a radical health education practice', *Radical Health Promotion*, 4. pp. 24–8.

AUERBACH, D. M. *et al* (1984) 'Cluster of cases of the Acquired Immune Deficiency Syndrome: Patients linked by sexual contact, *American Journal of Medicine*, 76. pp 487–92.

BEATTIE, A. (1986) 'Community development for health: From practice to theory', *Radical Health Promotion*, 4, pp. 12–18.

BMJ (1986) 'AIDS: Act now, don't pay later', *Editorial*, 9 August. p 348.

BURTON, S. *et al* (1986) 'AIDS information', *Lancet*, 8514, 2, pp 1040–1.

CDR (1986) 'Acquired Immune Deficiency Syndrome', *Communicable Diseases Report*, 86/31, July.

CLARITY COLLECTIVE (1985) *Taught not Caught: Strategies for Sex Education*, Wisbech, Learning Development Aids.

COWARD, R. (1987) 'Sex after AIDS', *New Internationalist*, March.

CRAIG, M. (1987) *Report on the AIDS training project*, Bristol, National Health Service Training Authority.

CRIBB, A. (1986) 'Politics and Health in the school curriculum' in RODMELL, S. and WATT, A. (Eds.) *The Politics of Health Education*, London, Routledge and Kegan Paul.

DHSS (1986) press release 86/244.

DICKSON, A. (1982) *A Woman in Your Own Right*, London, Quartet Books.

DICKSON, A. (1985) *The Mirror Within: A New Look at Sexuality*, London, Quartet Books.

DiCLEMENTE, R. *et al* (1986) 'Adolescents and AIDS: A survey of knowledge, attitudes and beliefs about AIDS in San Francisco', *American Journal of Public Health*, 76, 12, pp 1443–5.

DIXON, H. (1986) *Options for Change: A Staff Training Handbook on Personal Relationships and Sexuality for People with Mental Handicap*, London, FPA Education Unit.

DRAPER, P. *et al* (1980) 'Three types of health education', *British Medical Journal*, 16 August, pp. 493–5.

FRENCH, J. and ADAMS, L. (1986) 'From analysis to synthesis', *Health Education Journal*, 45, 2. pp. 71–4.

GALLO, R. *et al* (1985) 'The etiology of AIDS' in DE VITA, V. T. *et al* (Eds.) *AIDS: Etiology, Diagnosis, Treatment and Prevention*, Philadelphia, PA, Lippincott.

GATHERER, A. *et al* (1979) *Is Health Education Effective?*, London, Health Education Council.

GAZZARD, B. *et al* (1984) 'Clinical findings and serological evidence of HTLV-III infection in homosexual contacts of patients with AIDS and persistent generalized lymphadenopathy in London', *Lancet.*, 1 September, pp 480–3.

GELLAN, M. and ISON, C. (1986) 'Declining incidence of gonorrhoea in London: A response to fear of AIDS', *Lancet*, 8512, 2, p 920.

GREEN, J. (1986a) 'Counselling HTLV-III seropositives' in MILLER, D. *et al* (Eds.) *The Management of AIDS Patients*, Basingstoke, Macmillan.

GREEN, J. (1986b) 'Reduction of risk in high risk groups' in MILLER, D. *et al* (Eds.) *The Management of Patients with AIDS*, Basingstoke, Macmillan.

Guardian (1986) 'The scourge of doing nothing' 11 August.

HUMAN RIGHTS FOUNDATION (1984) *Demystifying Homosexuality: A Teaching Guide about Lesbians and Gay Men*, New York, Irvington.

INSTITUTE OF MEDICINE, NATIONAL ACADEMY OF SCIENCES (1987) *Confronting AIDS*, Washington, National Academy Press.

JOHNSON, H. and HO, P. (1985) 'The elusive etiology — Possible causes and pathogenesis of AIDS' in GONG, V. (Ed.) *Understanding AIDS*, Cambridge, Cambridge University Press.

LISCOMBE, H. (1985) 'The immunology of AIDS' in GONG (Ed.) *Understanding AIDS*, Cambridge, Cambridge University Press.

LUSSIER, R. (1984) 'The history of health education', in ROBINSON, L. and ALLES, W. (Eds.) *Health Education: Foundations for the Future*, Philadelphia, PA, Mosby.

MCKUSICK, L. *et al* (1985) 'AIDS and sexual behaviour reported by gay men in San Francisco', *American Journal of Public Health*, 75. 5. pp 493–6.

MILLER, C. (1987) 'AIDS — A city strategy', *Medicine in Society*, Spring. pp. 29–32.

MILLS, S. *et al* (1986) 'Public knowledge of AIDS and the DHSS advertisement campaign', *British Medical Journal*, 293, pp 1089–90.

MITCHELL, J. (1982) 'Looking after ourselves: An individual approach', *Journal of the Royal Society of Health*. 4.

MORAN, G. (1986) 'Radical health promotion: A role for local authorities?' in RODMELL, S. and WATT, A. (Eds.) *The Politics of Health Education*, London, Routledge and Kegan Paul.

NAIDOO, J. (1986) 'Limits to individualism' in RODMELL, S. and WATT, A. (Eds.) *The Politics of Health Education*, London, Routledge and Kegan Paul.

NUPE (1987) *NUPE Journal*, 3, p 9.

ORTLEB, C. (1985a) 'AIDSGATE goes to Albany — Jean Dodds and African swine fever', *New York Native*, 1 July. p 35.

ORTLEB, C. (1985b) 'New York State to test for African swine fever', *New York Native*, 15 July. p 6.

ORTLEB, C. (1985c) 'Antibodies to African swine fever found in city blood bank', *New York Native*, 30 September. p 14.

ORTLEB, C. (1986a) 'The AIDS explosion in Cuba', *New York Native*, 17 February, p 4.

ORTLEB, C. (1986b) 'Infected pork may cause AIDS', *New York Native*, 31 March, pp 4 and 7.

ORTLEB, C. (1986b) 'Pigs in Belle Glade test positive for HTLV-III', *New York Native*, 9 June. pp 8–9.

ORTLEB, C. (1986e) 'Belle Glade mystery deepens', *New York Native*, 9 June pp 8–9.

ORTLEB, C. (1986e) 'Belle glade mystery deepens', *New York Native*, 9 June pp 8–9.

ORTLEB, C. (1986f) 'The news from Haiti', *New York Native*, 18 August. p 4.

PARSONS, T. (1957) 'The distribution of power in American society', *World Politics*, 10, pp 123–43.

PATTON, C. (1985) *Sex and Germs: The Politics of AIDS*, Boston, MA, South End Press.

PINCHING, A. (1986) 'Immunology' in JONES, P. (Ed.) *Proceedings of the AIDS Conference 1986*, Ponteland, Intercept Books.

POLLOCK, S. (1985) 'Sex and the contraceptive act' in HOMANS, H. (Ed.) *The Sexual Politics of Reproduction*, Aldershot, Gower.

RICHARDSON, D. (1987) *Women and AIDS*, London, Pandora Press.

RODMELL, S. and WATT, A. (1986) *The Politics of Health Education*, London, Routledge and Kegan Paul.

SATOW, A. (1987) personal communication.

SHAW, N. and PALCO, L. (1986) 'Women and AIDS' in MCKUSICK, L. (Ed.) *What to Do about AIDS*, Los Angeles, CA, University of California Press.

SILIN, J. (1987) 'Dangerous knowledge', *Christopher Street*, 113, pp 34–40.

SILVERMAN, M. (1986) 'What we have learned' in MCKUSICK, L. (Ed.) *What to Do about AIDS*, Los Angeles, CA, University of California Press.

SONNABEND, J. *et al* (1983) 'Acquired Immune Deficiency Syndrome: Opportunistic infections and malignancies in male homosexuals', *Journal of the American Medical Association*, 249. pp 2370–4.

SPENCE, C. (1986) *AIDS: Time to Reclaim Our Power*, London, Lifestory.

SZIROM, T. and DYSON, S. (1986) *Greater Expectations: A Source Book for Working with Girls and Young Women*, Wisbech, Learning Development Aids.

TATCHELL, P. (1986) *AIDS: A Guide to Survival*, London, Gay Men's Press.

WATT, A. (1986) 'Community health education: A time for caution?' in RODMELL, S. and WATT, A. (Eds.) *The Politics of Health Education*. London, Routledge and Kegan Paul.

WEBER, J. *et al* (1986) 'Factors affecting seropositivity to HTLV-III/LAV and progression of the disease in partners of patients with AIDS', *Lancet*, 14 May, pp. 1179–1181.

WELLS, N. (1986) *The AIDS Virus — Forecasting its Impact*, London, Office of Health Economics.

WORLD HEALTH ORGANIZATION (1986) 'Health promotion — A discussion document on the concept and principles', supplement to Europe News 3, Copenhagen, WHO Regional Office for Europe.

WORLD HEALTH ORGANIZATION (1986) 'Report of the meeting on educational strategies for the prevention and control of AIDS', Geneva, WHO, AIDS/CPA. 86, 4.

10
Visual AIDS — Advertising Ignorance

Simon Watney

On the last Sunday of 1986, *The Observer* informed its readers with a bracing mixture of ignorance and insensitivity that '1987 would be the second year of AIDS for Britain'.[1] It had evidently not occurred to journalist Nicholas Wapshott that ever since the HIV virus was identified in 1983, every year has been a 'Year of AIDS' — as he so crassly put it — for the gay population of the UK. That is, for the one to two million gay men who have been living through these terrible times with varying degrees of anxiety and fear, courage and dignity. Wapshott may observe that 'AIDS is not a gay plague, nor ever was', but his words ring hollow in the context of his metaphor of unexploded bombs for those infected by the virus, and sickeningly hypocritical cant about the need for 'sympathy and understanding for those trapped by their own proclivities'. Such euphemistically stilted language makes it painfully clear that AIDS is still being handled right across the media with all the most up to date medical, psychiatric and sociological resources of the late nineteenth century.

According to Wapshott's standardized version of recent events, 'Norman Fowler emerges as an unlikely hero in this miserable story'. It is certainly a miserable tale, but if Mr. Fowler has been heroic it is only in forcing the present government to recognize something of the full enormity of an epidemic which the rest of Europe faced up to some years ago. The official campaign which Mr. Fowler has launched suggests that government understanding of AIDS remains lamentably defective. 1986 was undoubtedly the first 'Year of AIDS' as far as British politicians of all persuasions were concerned. What this means in simple terms is that thousands will now inevitably die, as the direct result of prudery, moralism and an exaggerated faith in the medical profession's ability to find a cure or vaccine for HIV infection, aided and abetted by the resounding silence of the entire British party political system.

Inciting Ignorance

In New York City, AIDS is now the leading killer of women aged between 25 and 29, and is reckoned to become 'the leading cause of death of all women of child bearing age in New York by 1988'.[2] In Britain the number of newly-reported cases doubled between October and November 1986, bringing the total to 599, of whom 296 were already dead. This total included seventeen women, two babies, eleven patients infected by blood transfusions, and twenty-two haemophiliacs. The Centers for Disease Control in Atlanta, Georgia reported a total of 27,773 cases in the United States as of 17 November, of whom 15,597 were dead.[3] This was the grim backdrop against which the British government launched its first 'forceful' propaganda campaign 'to alert the public to the risk of AIDS'.[4] In the run-up to a critical General Election, AIDS was clearly the subject of massive political crisis management. It is therefore important to recall that the epidemiology of AIDS varies dramatically from country to country and from region to region. Thus in New York, more than 50 per cent of people with AIDS are black, Hispanic or Latino, whilst in London, like San Francisco, more than 90 per cent are gay. This is only to note a commonplace of medical history, that all epidemics emerge in specific localized constituencies. Blaming these constituencies for their affliction is as cruel and stupid as it would be to blame teenage mothers for getting pregnant when a national survey reveals that only 3.9 per cent of 649 women having abortions had received any contraception advice at school.[5] What remains so particularly shocking and obnoxious about the treatment of AIDS in the UK is the way in which the very social group most devastated by the disease has simply been left to suffer and die.

Thus the Terrence Higgins Trust, until recently the only voluntary organization providing information and counselling services to gay men and the rest of the population, has had to struggle along with a mere £100,000 pa of public assistance. The Trust has needed a minimum of £250,000 pa for its educational work and support services for people with AIDS, and the shortfall has been raised by intensive fund-raising amongst gay men. And all along the line its activities have been hampered by doctors and politicians holding the purse-strings, who have refused to support the production and distribution of explicit safer sex materials for gay men.

Safer sex videos like the New York gay men's health crisis' *Chance of a Lifetime* are currently banned in Britain by ludicrous censorship laws, and until HM Customs dropped their charges against London's *Gay's The Word* bookshop in the summer of 1986 none of the leading American or

European gay newspapers containing the most up to date information and debate about AIDS were available in the UK. They could not be safely imported. Hence the all but incredible story of how the government's own Chief Medical Officer had to have copies of *The Advocate* and *New York Native* smuggled into England in diplomatic bags to avoid the possibility of their seizure as the current AIDS campaign was first being drawn up.[6]

As long ago as August 1983 the British *Medical News* recommended gay men start using condoms as a matter of routine sexual practice,[7] and more recently the respected American medical correspondent Ann Guidici Fettner has pointed out that 'AIDS education should have been started the moment it was realized that the disease is sexually transmitted'.[8] This is precisely what voluntary organizations like the Terrence Higgins Trust have been saying all along. But as long as AIDS was perceived as a 'gay plague' the entire problem was only calculated in terms of the possible 'leakage' from affected groups to the 'general public', from which gay men are evidently categorically excluded. The belated recognition that it is not 'just' prostitutes and drug-users and 'queers' who are at risk, but even those living in the Tory shires, explains much of the current campaign. Thus an advert appeared in many magazines at Christmas 1986, spelling out the word 'AIDS' in seasonal wrapping paper, with the accompanying question 'How many people will get it for Christmas?'. Another advert conveys the message that 'Your next sexual partner could be that very special person', framed inside a heart like a Valentine card, beneath with we read the supplement, — 'The one that gives you AIDS'. The official line is clearly anti-sex, drawing on an assumed rhetoric concerning 'promiscuity' as the supposed 'cause' of AIDS, in order to terrorize people into monogamy. But monogamy is no more intrinsically safe than any other kind of sex, unless precautions are taken. Mortal fears are being whipped up, as if sexuality were entirely within the control of rational consciousness, and as if sexual desire were a tap with just two simple positions, on and off.

Still more problematic was the ubiquitous series of posters which appeared all over Britain in early 1987, their messages seemingly carved into granite-like tomb-stones. Thus we read the solemn injunction 'AIDS: DON'T DIE OF IGNORANCE', with the secondary advice that 'Anyone can get it, gay or straight, male or female. Already 30,000 people are infected'. The same poster continued, 'At the moment the infection is mainly confined to relatively small groups of people in this country. But it is spreading'. Something extraordinary is going on here. On the one hand the government appears to acknowledge the actual diversity of sexual identities in the modern world, yet at another this is evidently not the case since we were simultaneously intended to dismiss all thought of the vast majority of people with AIDS as members of 'relatively small groups of people'. The poster also peddled a mischievous implication of responsibility onto people with AIDS as if they had somehow set out to contract it by ignoring advice and information which has never been widely available. It also cynically looked entirely over the heads of all those most immediately affected by the epidemic. Apart from lesbians and gay men, which other social group with almost 800 dead and dying could have been so casually erased from all public consideration?

'AIDS IS NOT PREJUDICED: IT CAN KILL ANYONE' screamed another poster, this time with the sub-heading 'It's true more men than women have AIDS. But this does not mean it is a homosexual disease. It isn't'. Here could be found the astounding implication either that there *are* viruses which consciously select their victims, motivated by sexual desire, or that some diseases are the intrinsic properties of gay men. There is of course no such thing as a virus which only affects men *or* women, but medical facts are irrelevant here, since what the poster is actually saying is that it doesn't matter if you *are* prejudiced, as long as you don't make the mistake of thinking that AIDS is 'only' killing off the queers.

Yet another poster proclaims that 'THE LONGER YOU BELIEVE AIDS ONLY INFECTS OTHERS, THE FASTER IT'LL SPREAD'. Whilst the 'you' addressed here was at least open to all readers to identify with, there was still no information and advice — beyond the totally incorrect implication that AIDS is itself infectious. This inability to distinguish between AIDS and the HIV virus was typical of a campaign which was evidently not educational in any useful sense, but which aimed only to frighten and alarm as many people as possible.

The worst poster simply asked 'AIDS: HOW BIG DOES IT HAVE TO GET BEFORE YOU TAKE NOTICE?'. It was, however, far from clear quite what we were expected to 'take notice' of, beyond the poster itself, which again suggests that the campaign was largely diversionary, giving the impression that the government is doing something about AIDS and has the epidemic in hand. The question which we should be asking some five years into the epidemic is how big did it have to get before *they* took any notice. The folly of the entire campaign was its total failure to talk to people in any but the most abstract and over-generalized terms. We thus still face the nightmarish situation of an epidemic running out of control, under a government and opposition which are totally unable to acknowledge or address the actual social and sexual diversity of the society which they purport to represent.

The same obituary graphics are used on the front of the leaflet recently distributed to every household in Britain. Like the posters, it was drawn up without any consultation whatsoever with the Terrence Higgins Trust, or any organization with direct experience of AIDS educational work. To add insult to injury the Terrence Higgins Trust's telephone number was placed on the leaflet without permission, and in belated recognition of the fact that it would be swamped with calls the government agreed to install a number of extra telephone lines. Whilst the leaflet offers a lot of straightforward and helpful information, it nonetheless proceeds from the statement that AIDS is 'not just a homosexual disease'. This is a shocking and disgraceful statement, and if anyone still doubts that gay men are officially regarded *in their entirety* as a disposable community, they need look no further. In 1983, when there were less than 3000 recorded cases of AIDS in the United States, Richard Goldstein wrote that 'for heterosexuals to act as if AIDS were a threat to everyone demeans the anxiety of gay men to act as if we're all going to die, demeans the anguish of those who are actually ill'.[9] His message is as timely as ever. Millions of pounds have been squandered in a face-saving exercise which has directed its crude loud-hailing machinery at nobody in particular, least of all towards those who are most in need of a positive health education programme. How could this be otherwise from a government which is profoundly hostile to sex education as such, and which in all other circumstances regards gay men only as the target for ever increasingly punitive legislation, prosecution, and surveillance?

Diversity and Desire

The government's 1987 AIDS campaign offered no correction whatsoever to the chorus of stubbornly opinionated ignorance which hitherto had constituted most AIDS commentary in the UK. In the absence of a strong affirmative national gay culture, British gays are especially vulnerable to AIDS. This is why the didactic call not 'to die of ignorance' is so insufferable, since gay men have been so efficiently kept in ignorance of AIDS throughout the 1980s by courtesy of this government and its various agencies. British gay culture is fragmentary and atomized, lacking even the most elementary civil rights consciousness, unable even to organize a proper national newspaper. In this respect we are victimized by the direct legacy of centuries of British homophobia, active at every level of culture and the state in ways which clearly mark Britain apart from the rest of Europe, as is reflected in a host of archaic and fundamentally undemocratic legislations.

The government's AIDS initiative was no more than an extension of the familiar public agenda for 'thinking' AIDS, something which has proved so stubbornly resistant to the actual complexity of issues raised by the epidemic. Couched within a discourse whose words are sticky with blood-lust, hatred and thinly-veiled contempt for the thousands of sick and dying, it offered a heady brew of racism, mysogyny and homophobia, which speaks volumes about the real moral condition of contemporary Britain. That socialists and feminists alike have so totally failed to grasp the implications of AIDS for the future political management of these islands is particularly regrettable. We are all living through a catastrophe which has been systematically denied the status of a natural disaster, let alone a tragedy. This terrible epidemic should teach us once and for all that if our species has any worth or beauty it lies in its diversity, and our capacity to embrace and celebrate all our variously consenting states of desire. And if in these dreadful times we should wish somewhat to alleviate the pain of our losses — of freedoms and of friends — then we might think of AIDS as a monstrously ironic means to that end.

Notes

1 WAPSHOTT, N. (1986) 'New morality and the sexual time bomb', *The Observer*, 28 December.

2 D'ADESKY, A. C. (1986) 'AIDS: A serious threat to women', *New York Native*, 187.

3 *New York Native* (1986) 189, p 23.

4 'Cabinet AIDS drive aimed at all homes', *The Guardian*, 12 November 1986.

5 'Schools leave girls in the dark about sex', *The Guardian*, 2 March 1987.

6 'People at large', *The Guardian*, 18 March 1986.

7 'Homosexuals advised to use condoms to prevent AIDS', *Medical News*, 15 August 1983.

8 GIUDICI FETTNER, A. (1986) 'Is the CDC dying of AIDS?', *Village Voice*, 7 October, p 16.

9 GOLDSTEIN, R. (1983) 'Heartsick: Fear and loving in the gay community', *Village Voice*, 28 June, p 12.

Author Index

Subject Index